Epilepsy in Other Brain Diseases

A substantial proportion of patients with other brain diseases like stroke, traumatic brain injury, and dementia will develop epilepsy. This book provides a clear and concise guide to the epidemiology and clinical research on epilepsy as it occurs in the context of other brain diseases.

A better and more detailed understanding of the diseases related to the brain following decades of advances in neuroimaging, pathology, and neurophysiology have led to new insights into mechanisms leading to epilepsy. Advances in research on epilepsy in one brain disease are known to lead to an improved understanding of epilepsy in others. Advances in neurological care have resulted in patients with stroke, tumors, or infections surviving longer, with ensuing demands for long-term treatment, including epilepsy.

A key message across the different chapters in the book is that epilepsy in other brain diseases should be managed just as ambitiously as any other epilepsy. Neurologists treating patients with brain disease will find this book accessible and practical. It will ensure a deeper understanding of acquired epilepsy among clinicians.

Epilepsy in Other Brain Diseases
A Guide to Diagnosis and Management

Johan Zelano

Professor of Neurology, University of Gothenburg
and Sahlgrenska University Hospital

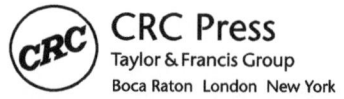

CRC Press
Taylor & Francis Group
Boca Raton London New York

CRC Press is an imprint of the
Taylor & Francis Group, an **informa** business

Designed cover image: Shutterstock

First edition published 2025
by CRC Press
2385 NW Executive Center Drive, Suite 320, Boca Raton FL 33431

and by CRC Press
4 Park Square, Milton Park, Abingdon, Oxon, OX14 4RN

CRC Press is an imprint of Taylor & Francis Group, LLC

ISBN: 9781032817941 (hbk)
ISBN: 9781032815213 (pbk)
ISBN: 9781003501404 (ebk)

DOI: 10.1201/9781003501404

Typeset in Times LT STD
by Apex CoVantage, LLC

To my patients.

Contents

About the Author

Johan Zelano is Professor of neurology at the University of Gothenburg and Sahlgrenska University Hospital, Sweden. His research group focuses on acquired epilepsies and runs a research program comprising population-wide studies on epilepsy in stroke, multiple sclerosis, dementia, brain infections and trauma, and clinical studies on epilepsy biomarkers. Professor Zelano is past president of the Swedish Neurological Society and member of the board of the Swedish Epilepsy Society. He has been a speaker on acquired epilepsy at the three last European congresses of epileptology. In 2019, he cofounded a scientific conference on epilepsy after stroke (Seizures and Stroke), which since 2023 has been transformed into a meeting on all symptomatic and structural epilepsies and attracts participants from all over Europe. He has been associate editor of the scientific journal *Acta Neurologica Scandinavica* and currently serves in that role for *Epilepsia Open*. He maintains an epilepsy practice at Sahlgrenska University Hospital and is involved in undergraduate and graduate education at the University of Gothenburg.

Preface

Approximately half of all cases of epilepsy are caused by another brain disease, and such acquired epilepsy is encountered throughout the health care system. Many management questions are often faced by non-epilepsy specialists in a range of medical specialties. This book offers an introduction to the field as well as an overview of current research. Hopefully, the book will also be of interest to preclinical scientists doing epilepsy research and wanting to understand more about the human condition.

The book is short in order to be accessible. There are fictive case descriptions in each chapter, entirely made up by me. Any resemblance to actual persons is a coincidence. The book also describes research discussing off-label treatments and should not be interpreted as a clinical guideline or recommendation. The aim has been to provide an overview of a clinical field; such an overview can hopefully help clinicians develop a deeper understanding of acquired epilepsy—which will in turn allow better care of patients.

The level of evidence is often low in epilepsy, and the heterogeneity among patients with epilepsy in another brain disease has been an obstacle for gathering meaningful clinical data. Fortunately, with big data the situation seems to be changing, and there is now hope for more personalized treatment in the next few years. Nonetheless, for many of the epilepsies discussed in the book we have insufficient information about prognosis and clinical courses. Here, I hope that the book can contribute by pointing out important questions for future research.

The book has been very interesting to write. There is a lot of impressive work being done by researchers and clinicians to try to understand, treat, and in the future perhaps prevent epilepsy in other brain disorders. Thanks to their efforts, we can treat our patients increasingly better.

Johan Zelano
Gothenburg
September 29, 2024

Introduction

1

1.1 WHY A BOOK ON EPILEPSY IN OTHER BRAIN DISEASES?

There are several reasons for compiling a brief introduction to epilepsy in other brain diseases. A better and more detailed understanding of the diseases of the brain following decades of advances in neuroimaging, pathology, and neurophysiology have led to new insights into mechanisms leading to epilepsy. As will hopefully become clear throughout the following chapters, advances in research on epilepsy in one brain disease leads to a better understanding of epilepsy in others. Furthermore, neurological care has advanced. Patients with stroke, tumors, or infections survive longer, with ensuing demands for adequate treatment of sequelae like epilepsy. Finally, research is accumulating on epilepsy in specific brain diseases, which gradually builds a foundation for personalized medicine; patients can increasingly be advised and treated based on data from representative populations. At the same time, a holistic perspective is also needed—which is another reason for a book on epilepsy in other brain diseases. There are commonalities in pathogenesis as well as management and much to be gained from an integrated approach. This book attempts to use both perspectives for a better understanding and ultimately treatment of patients with epilepsy in other brain diseases.

Naturally, there are limitations. This book focuses on the quantitatively dominating brain diseases: stroke, infections, traumatic brain injury, dementia, and the most common brain tumors. These are common causes of new-onset seizures and frequently encountered in emergency care, internal medicine, or general neurology (Figure 1.1). Immune-mediated epilepsies are also included, because it is a field that has advanced our understanding of epileptogenesis in recent years and unraveled disease processes that are probably relevant in most if not all other epilepsies, at least the acquired ones. In contrast, rarer brain diseases like encephalopathies with presentation in childhood, tumors encountered in surgical work-up of refractory epilepsy, or metabolic epilepsies with a genetic origin are not extensively discussed. These are interesting topics but highly specialized and outside the scope of this book.

DOI: 10.1201/9781003501404-1

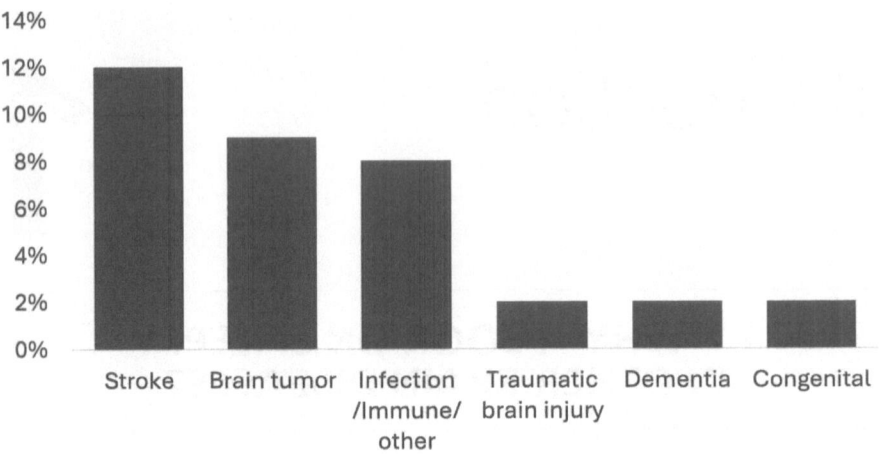

FIGURE 1.1 Proportion of different etiologies in new-onset unprovoked seizures in Stockholm, Sweden.[1]

1.2 NEGLECTED EPILEPSIES?

Epilepsy is a heterogeneous condition. The predisposition of an individual for unprovoked seizures can be the result of many pathophysiological processes, genetic as well as such acquired throughout life. The epilepsy incidence curve (Figure 1.2) clearly illustrates the sharp rise in epilepsy that occurs in middle age and after, reflecting the impact of stroke and other brain damage accumulated by ageing. It is therefore somewhat surprising that epilepsy arising in other brain diseases did not attract much research interest for a long time. For instance, studies on the global burden of disease focus mainly on genetic/idiopathic epilepsies, despite epilepsy from infections and cerebrovascular disease being more common.[2] As a consequence, epilepsy in other brain disorders had attracted relatively limited research interest until the last decades. A realization among researchers, decision makers, and research funders that acquired epilepsy accounts for a large and increasing proportion of epilepsy in most countries, as well as patient/caregiver demands, have probably all been important factors driving the increased research efforts of the last decades.

Lack of proper scientific tools are perhaps another explanation for the earlier low academic interest in epilepsy in other brain diseases. Patients with stroke, dementia, or traumatic brain injury are typically not followed by doctors studying epilepsy and therefore perhaps less visible as research subjects. Before digital communication and infrastructure like registers, studying epilepsy of a single etiology was difficult. The shift started with increasing sizes of data sets, a development clearly illustrated by the larger studies on poststroke epilepsy that started to emerge after 2010, confirming that seizures are a very common stroke sequalae.[3,4]

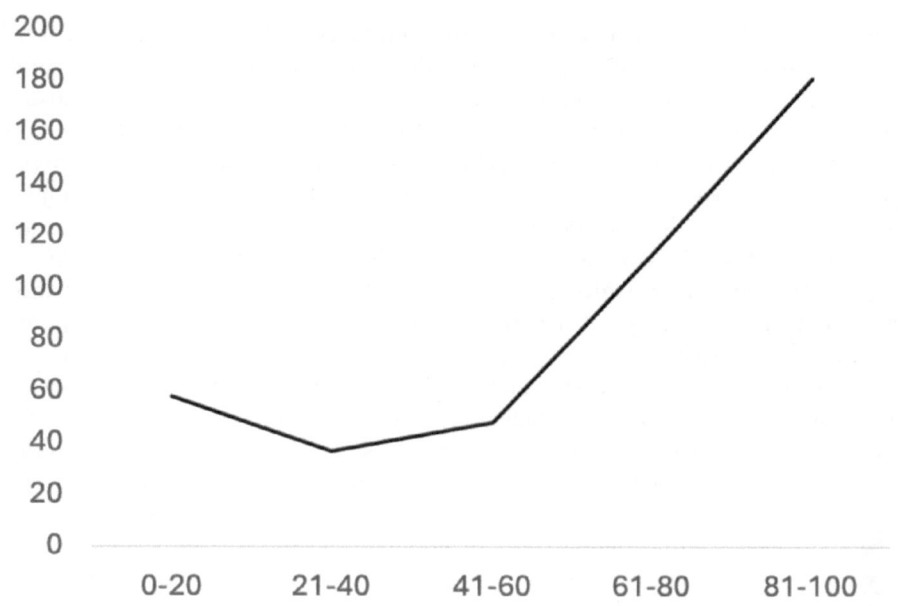

FIGURE 1.2 Incidence of epilepsy in Sweden 2016–17 in different age groups n/100.000 person years.[5]

Since epilepsy in other brain diseases is common, there has naturally been much clinical knowledge and expert opinions among neurologists, but compilation of big enough datasets to allow meaningful stratification by etiology has become common only with the advance of big data tools. A clear example is the Rochester epilepsy epidemiology project, which was an early effort to stratify epilepsy by etiology in analyses of risk factors and prognosis.[6] The project has contributed greatly to our understanding of epilepsy in other brain diseases, but from today's perspective it contained relatively few participants in each etiology in different age groups.

1.3 ADVANCES THROUGH STRATIFICATION BY ETIOLOGY

With some exceptions, patients with epilepsy in other brain diseases have been studied under the broad umbrella term of focal epilepsy. This approach has had advantages, but also drawbacks. Among the benefits are great conditions for studies of efficacy of newer antiseizure medications (ASM). Focal epilepsy has been the go-to epilepsy for sponsors of clinical trials, and there are now over 25 drugs registered for treatment of focal epilepsy in Europe and the US. Among the drawbacks are that the enormous heterogeneity of focal epilepsy makes it difficult to use data from such clinical trials for personalized tailored treatments. The study population are also often younger than the average person with epilepsy acquired in another brain disease. There is also heterogeneity within patients with epilepsy in another brain disease. The relative importance of different side effects, teratogenicity, drug–drug interactions, and prognosis obviously differs between a young woman with epilepsy after traumatic brain injury or autoimmune encephalitis and an older man with epilepsy after ischemic stroke caused by atrial fibrillation. In summary, composite studies on all types of focal epilepsy will not provide guidance on which drug is best for which patient. With the advance of personalized medicine, patients rightly expect to be treated based on data from representative patient groups.

Fortunately, the situation is changing. Advances in epidemiology, genetics, neurophysiology, and neuroimaging made it clear that to be able to draw clinically meaningful conclusions from results, epilepsy must also be studied according to etiology. Meanwhile, advances in immunology led to discovery of autoimmune causes of seizures, better brain tumor pathology led to recognition of differences in seizure prevalence and prognosis in different types of gliomas, and so on. The development with more focus on the cause of epilepsy is most clearly illustrated by the 2017 ILAE classification of epilepsies in which etiology is one of the important axes (Figure 1.3).[7]

As a result, our knowledge of epilepsy in other brain diseases is advancing on many fronts. The advantages are clear with regards to providing patients with personalized prognostication, unravelling of disease-specific pathological processes, and quantification of the impact on quality of life of patients as well as societal costs. These advances fill a substantial need. For most if not all populations described in the following chapters, there is a substantial knowledge gap on important management issues.

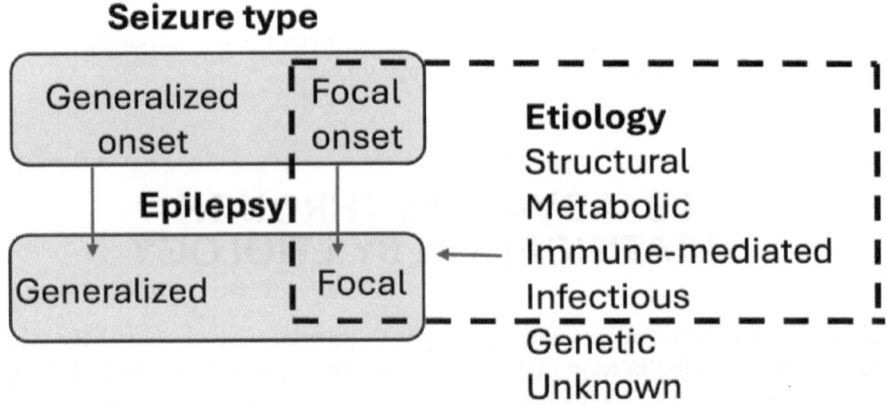

FIGURE 1.3 The ILAE classification categorizes epilepsy by seizure type and etiology. Epilepsy in other brain diseases generally causes focal-onset seizures and therefore focal epilepsies (dashed).

1.4 EPIDEMIOLOGY CONTRIBUTIONS

Big data like Scandinavian population-wide registers and US claims data have contributed to a greater understanding of exactly how common epilepsy is in various brain diseases. Out of adults with stroke in Sweden, about 7% will go on develop epilepsy.[8] The risk of epilepsy is about 4% for all traumatic brain injury,[9] 4% in dementia,[10] 6% after brain infections,[11] and 3.5% for multiple sclerosis.[12] There is substantial variation within these categories that seems linked to severity and cortical affliction of the brain injury; the epilepsy risk is 13% in severe traumatic brain injury compared to 2.6% after mild,[9] 5.5% in secondary progressive MS compared to 3% in the relapsing remitting form,[12] and 30% after brain abscesses compared to just 4% after bacterial meningitis.[11]

Another epidemiological insight is that with ageing populations, acquired epilepsy is becoming a greater proportion of all epilepsy. Epilepsy is becoming a disease of the elderly and will remain so in the coming decades. This means that vascular risk factors and management of epilepsy in the context of comorbidities that are common in higher age will be more important in all epilepsy.[13] Structural and metabolic etiologies already account for more than 40% of prevalent epilepsy in Scandinavia/northern Europe.[14]

The epidemiology of symptomatic epilepsy today reflects the outcomes of underlying brain disorders of yesterday. Because of improved treatments, it is possible that future studies will show decreased risk of epilepsy after stroke, multiple sclerosis, and autoimmune encephalitis. Hopefully, this will lead to a better understanding on how to reduce the risk of epilepsy in other brain diseases as well. Improvements in the treatment of Alzheimer's disease and traumatic brain injury may result in similar changes in epilepsy risk in these conditions in the future. Finally, epidemiological surveillance can help our understanding of the contribution of different etiologies to the global burden of epilepsy in other brain diseases.

1.5 NEED FOR IMPROVED MANAGEMENT

Clinical research on epilepsy in other brain diseases has also made it clear that clinical management is not always optimal and that some patient groups could be cared for better. For instance, poststroke epilepsy is often described as easy to treat in older literature and in many randomized trials, where nearly 80% achieve seizure freedom. Retrospective studies, however, show that many patients with poststroke epilepsy are not seizure free. This could reflect that poststroke epilepsy is not very easy to treat in all patients and that the randomized trials with the highest seizure freedom rates may have had some selection bias (smaller stroke, long latency, etc.) because researchers tend to recruit those likely to finish the trial. An alternative explanation could be that the trials are actually right and that routine clinical care fails to deliver seizure freedom to the degree that is biologically achievable.

There are other indirect indications that epilepsy in other brain diseases is not optimally managed. Standard-of-care items like side effects and seizure situation are not always addressed if patients are followed mainly for another condition like multiple sclerosis or stroke and not seen by doctors trained in epilepsy.[15,16] Fortunately, there seems to be an increased awareness on the importance of good epilepsy care if patents also have another brain disease. The European guidelines on dementia, for instance, underlines the importance of good epilepsy treatment, as do expert opinions on brain tumor–related epilepsy.[17,18]

1.6 HOW TO TREAT EPILEPSY IN OTHER BRAIN DISEASES

A key message across the different chapters in the book is that epilepsy in other brain diseases should be managed just as ambitiously as any other epilepsy. That means careful assessment of risk of recurrence after a first seizure, tailored selection of a first ASM, increases in dose until seizure freedom or intolerable side effects, therapy revision if needed, and follow-up with a particular focus on side effects, safety, and psychiatric comorbidities (Figure 1.4). Comorbidities and concomitant medications frequently need to be considered. Any physician instigating ASM therapy in a person with epilepsy can contribute greatly to the quality of care by ensuring that the patient will receive follow-up and that someone will inquire about side effects or continued seizures. All too often, patients with epilepsy after stroke, after traumatic brain injury, or in dementia are started on an ASM and simply not followed up from an epilepsy perspective.

The most common first ASMs in focal epilepsies in Europe are probably lamotrigine, levetiracetam, oxcarbazepine, carbamazepine, or lacosamide, but alternative monotherapies may include topiramate, zonisamide, eslicarbazepine, valproate, or phenytoin.[19] In addition to patient factors and side effect sensitivity, local availability, regulatory guidelines, treatment traditions, cost, and restrictions on use in women of childbearing age are other factors that have influenced prescribers' choices and therefore the observational literature. For instance, there are strict restrictions on the use of topiramate and valproate in women of childbearing age. The fortunate development of many new ASMs means that there are many treatment options, and with more research there will hopefully be more evidence in the future on how to best use the wider therapeutic arsenal.

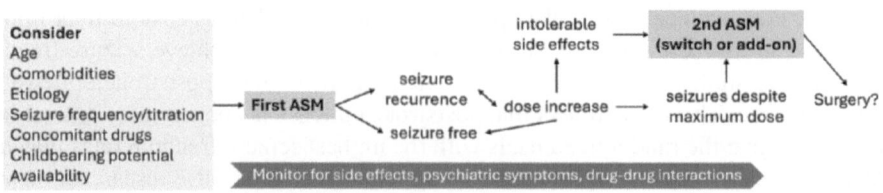

FIGURE 1.4 Outline of epilepsy treatment. The aim is seizure freedom without or with only minimal side effects.

1.7 EPILEPTOGENESIS: COMMON CLUES

Epileptogenesis refers to the alteration of brain networks and other changes that lead to a predisposition for unprovoked seizures. It is a conceptual term, since these processes are often unknown and multifactorial. Advances in neuropathology, genetics, fluid biomarkers, and imaging allow greater access to the brain and has furthered our understanding. Common clues are beginning to emerge if one regards epilepsy in several brain diseases alongside one another (Table 1.1).

In all brain diseases, a greater injury is linked to a higher epilepsy risk. In distinct etiologies like brain infections, traumatic brain injury, and stroke, more extensive brain damage and cortical lesion carries the greatest risk. Hemorrhage seems to increase the risk further, perhaps through higher blood–brain barrier permeability or inflammation. In more insidious processes like dementia or multiple sclerosis, greater accumulation of damage, often measured as disability, increases the risk of epilepsy.

Another pattern that emerges is that the risk of epilepsy seems to follow a similar temporal pattern across different etiologies, at least after brain diseases with a definable onset like traumatic brain injury, stroke, and infection. The risk is highest in the first year, followed by a slightly lower risk in the second, and a lower but still above-normal risk after that. This indicates that in most individuals the alterations of epileptogenesis take some time. The interval overlaps with periods of plasticity after stroke and traumatic brain injury, suggesting that remodeling of neuronal networks could be a major factor. The first years also constitute the most prominent period of gliosis and neuroinflammation, which are strong contenders as processes contributing to epileptogenesis. Inflammation is detected in all brain diseases related to epilepsy, and upregulation of IL-1beta, TNF, and IL-6 seem among the most often discovered mediators. Which components of the neuroinflammatory response are specific to epilepsy is not known, but given that inflammation seems involved in most brain diseases it will be exciting to follow the development of potential antiepileptogenic therapies based on targets in neuroinflammation cascades. To date, most antiepileptogenesis studies have involved antiseizure medications, but such trials have been largely negative.

Genetics are another important common factor across epilepsy in other brain diseases. After traumatic brain injury and stroke, discussed in chapters 2 and 3,

TABLE 1.1   Common Factors in Epileptogenesis across Different Brain Diseases

Greater and cortical injury increases the risk
Temporal course—greatest risk in the first year
Acute symptomatic seizures, particularly status epilepticus, increases the risk
Inflammation
Genetic vulnerability

respectively, there is a slightly higher risk of epilepsy in patients with first-degree relatives with epilepsy. The risk is not elevated to an extent that suggests a major interaction between the insult and familial epilepsy risk, but at the same time, genetic variants have been identified that seem to increase the risk of poststroke epilepsy. These seemingly conflicting results may perhaps be explained by developments in the study of polygenic risk score, and the case for genetic contributions to at least some cases of epilepsy in other brain diseases is growing.[20] A possible future development is a better genetic risk assessment than the current practice (which is mainly asking about a first-degree relative with epilepsy). Actual genetic testing may form the basis for risk stratification in future clinical work-up of first seizures and supplement injury characteristics in risk assessment and decisions on the need for monitoring or future antiepileptogenic treatment.

The most recent advances in studies of epileptogenesis in humans have probably occurred in the fields of autoimmune encephalitis and brain tumors. As discussed in chapter 5, antibodies of different subclasses have different potential to cause epilepsy, which can be linked to distinct inflammatory responses. In fact, a substantial proportion of patients with autoimmune encephalitis do not seem to develop epilepsy once the inflammation has subsided, raising the issue of whether their seizures during the encephalitis really reflect epilepsy at all or an extended period of acute symptomatic seizures. In brain tumors, several epileptogenesis mechanisms seems to be at work, including inflammation and remodeling of brain networks, but also processes that are distinct to specific tumor types, like expulsion of glutamate or formation of pseudosynapses between tumor and neurons. The genetics of brain tumors are influential in determining epilepsy risk. Many mechanisms seem shared across etiologies (Figure 1.5).

Although we have many more clues, there is still much we do not understand about epileptogenesis, and the concept of latency from insult to epilepsy may be an

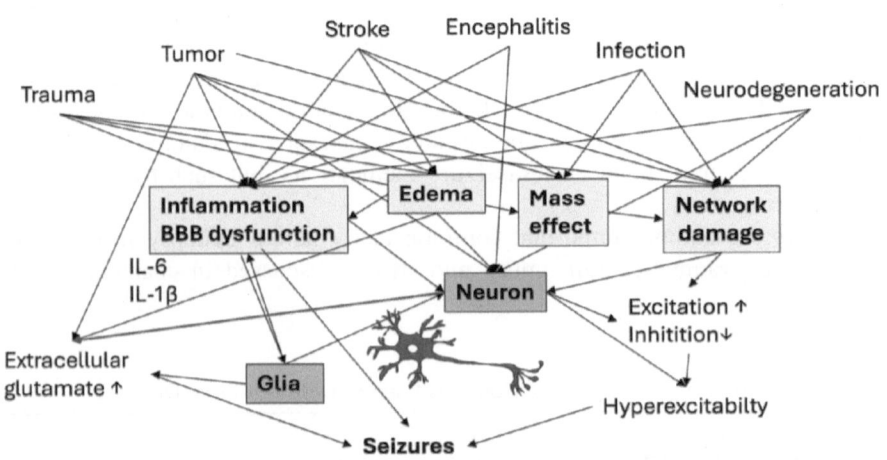

FIGURE 1.5 Epileptogenic mechanisms in other brain diseases work from tissue to cellular levels. Many are probably shared between different brain diseases.

oversimplification. For instance, acute symptomatic seizures at the onset of a brain disease, epileptiform activity on early EEG, or status epilepticus at the onset of a brain disorder are associated with an increased risk of subsequent epilepsy.

1.8 THE RISK OF MISDIAGNOSIS WITH A WIDER EPILEPSY DEFINITION

In 2014 the ILAE renewed the epilepsy definition by attaching a practical definition of epilepsy to the preexisting conceptual one. The new definition allows a diagnosis of epilepsy in the following cases: "One unprovoked (or reflex) seizure and a probability of further seizures similar to the general recurrence risk (above 60%) after two unprovoked seizures, occurring over the next 10 years."[21] Previous stroke is singled out as clinical circumstance where a diagnosis can be motivated after a first remote seizure, because of the high recurrence risk demonstrated in several studies, including an often cited study from Minnesota, with stroke being the most common etiology.[22]

As will become evident in the following chapters, the knowledge on recurrence risk in other brain disorders is far less extensive than that after stroke. Prior brain insults or abnormal brain imaging increase the risk of seizure recurrence about two-fold, but a proportion of patients with a first seizure and previous brain disease will not develop epilepsy.[23] The ILAE is clearly aware of the danger of a wider diagnosis and emphasizes that epilepsy should not be diagnosed after a first seizure in the absence of clear information on a >60% recurrence risk. The definition also states that "a single seizure plus a lesion" does not satisfy criteria for epilepsy.[21] This is currently the clinically most judicious approach. Misdiagnosis of epilepsy can have devastating consequences with ensuing stigma, costs, delayed search for alternative explanations, and unnecessary treatment with ASMs.[24] Relying on just one event for an epilepsy diagnosis also increases the risk of misdiagnosis based on non-epileptic events or because of acute symptomatic seizures being mislabeled as remote. Uncertainty is a poor basis for a life-altering diagnosis like epilepsy. Two seizures still seems like the most robust indicator of epilepsy for most patients, but this may change with more data allowing better predictions. Alternatively, new ASMs with fewer side effects may shift the balance towards more patients being treated before formal diagnosis. In the future, perhaps intermediary steps like "probable epilepsy" will remove some of the problems with the current dichotomized situation.

The potential problem of misdiagnosis is greatest in preexisting brain disorders in which epilepsy is not that common. First seizures after mild traumatic brain injury, in early multiple sclerosis, or in newly diagnosed dementia[9,10,12] could sometimes be due to chance. Several authors point out the increased subjectivity of the new definition.[25,26] There seems to be substantial discordance among the neurologists when trying to diagnose epilepsy based on the 60% threshold in patients with previous brain diseases.

There has also been some critique of the threshold in the definition, saying that 60% is perhaps too low if the aim is to indicate a future seizure risk similar to that in the traditional definition relying on two unprovoked seizures.[26]

All chapters in the book have a section on estimating seizure recurrence risk. They will hopefully inform the reader about how little evidence exists for most clinical situations, but also about when epilepsy can be said to be present already after a single unprovoked seizure. Currently, the literature indicates that this can be the case if a first unprovoked seizure occurs in the first years after stroke or very severe traumatic brain injury, which is discussed in detail in chapters 2 and 3, respectively.

1.8.1 More Knowledge, Less Epilepsy?

The ILAE definition is meant to be filled with increasingly greater knowledge on recurrence risk in specific clinical situations, which will allow personalized estimates of recurrence risk and correct epilepsy diagnoses. Importantly, such developments will not just mean that more situations will be defined as epilepsy. The reverse is happening in immune-mediated epilepsies and some infections; in autoimmune encephalitis with antibodies against certain surface antigens, experts argue that many patients may in fact have acute symptomatic seizures during their entire disease course, and that epilepsy does not exist after immunotherapy. This is discussed further in chapter 5, but in these cases, the risk of misdiagnosing epilepsy is probably high. Similarly, there is a discussion in the field of neurocysticercosis (see chapter 4) that many seizures occurring during a particular cyst stage are acute symptomatic seizures but that patients are too indiscriminately diagnosed with epilepsy.

More data will in time hopefully allow better predictions. In the end, it is of course unsatisfactory that epilepsy is still diagnosed based on a statistical estimate of seizure recurrence risk. What is really needed are robust biomarkers of epileptogenesis. These are perhaps emerging at last; each chapter discusses what is known about epileptogenesis and research that is ongoing on its detection. There are also endeavors to try to combine epileptogenesis biomarker research across the different etiologies. One large systematic review looking for biomarkers of post-brain injury epileptogenesis found that 15 biomarkers in blood and seven in CSF have been described as associated with post-brain injury epilepsy.[27] These biomarkers (including IL-6 and IL-1β) were often related to inflammation.

It hardly needs pointing out that a diagnosis of epilepsy is not required for treatment with ASMs. Clinicians are often faced with situations in which the benefits of treatment outweigh the drawbacks. Some examples can include if a first seizure has been particularly severe or status epilepticus, if the risk of recurrence is high although not clearly above the threshold for diagnosis or the patient finds the risk unacceptable, and a multitude of other scenarios. Understanding that treatment of ASMs does not have to be supported by a diagnosis of epilepsy is probably key to avoiding communicating a level of certainty regarding recurrence risk that simply does not exist. The importance of patient involvement and shared decision-making cannot be stressed enough in successful epilepsy care.

1.9 NEW ASMs: WHAT DO WE KNOW AND WHAT DO THEY ADD?

There are currently over 20 ASMs registered for focal epilepsy, as monotherapy or add-on. Registration-purpose trials demonstrate effectiveness against seizures and safety, but seldom have etiology-stratified cohorts. It does not seem feasible to recruit enough patients for etiology-stratified trials, so the wider inclusion criterium of focal epilepsy is likely to continue to be used. Even trials in poststroke epilepsy—which is relatively common—struggle to recruit more than about a hundred or so patients.[28] Trying something similar for post-traumatic or postencephalitic epilepsy seems very difficult. Some clinical guidance can be drawn from older participants in traditional randomized controlled trials (RCTs), but each etiology usually remains rare. Registration-purpose trials are also relatively short and therefore not informative about long-term effectiveness (Table 1.2).

Another problem with RCTs is that comparison of more than one ASM increases the number of patients needed, making very broad inclusion criteria the only way to finish studies. Although efforts like the SANAD trials[29,30] (large randomized open-label trials) have been informative—large RCTs may not be the only way to gather more data on which ASM works best in epilepsy in other brain diseases.

Indeed, observational studies are addressing the need for personalized data. In population-wide register data or large claims databases, several research groups across the world are trying to understand which ASM is best for patients with certain characteristics. Whether this big data approach will help remains to be seen, but initial results are promising and discussed in the following chapters. One problem is the clear publication bias towards Europe-US-Oceania in the big data literature. There are studies emerging from higher-income countries in Asia but large gaps for most of the developing world. With artificial intelligence on the rise, such a skewness of available training datasets may be problematic for inference of treatment outcomes that have a genetic component, such as side effect sensitivity to particular ASMs.

TABLE 1.2 Why Both Randomized and Observational Studies Are Needed in the Gathering of Evidence in Epilepsy in Other Brain Diseases

	RANDOMIZED TRIALS	*OBSERVATIONAL STUDIES*
Advantages	Very little bias, because of randomization High level of evidence	Big data allows studies of thousands of patients, also with rare etiologies of epilepsy Real-world outcomes in all patient groups Long-term follow-up
Disadvantages	Few patients Hard to recruit patients with other brain diseases, children, etc. Can often only compare at most a few ASMs Short follow-up	Vulnerable to bias

The emerging literature suggests that newer ASMs have important roles in the treatment of epilepsy in other brain diseases, by virtue of milder side effects and fewer drug–drug interactions with other medications. They also add a greater number of available ASMs to try in the pursuit of seizure freedom. For personalized treatment of epilepsy in other brain disease, evidence needs to be gathered from both randomized trials and observational studies.

CASE 1.1 Benefits of Therapy Revision

A 40-year-old female is referred for epilepsy therapy revision by primary care, since she is not seizure free. History and medical records from her country of birth indicate that she suffered a traumatic brain injury in her later teens and that seizures started a few months later. She describes feeling a strange but distinct sensation, cannot speak, and sometimes falls down. The larger episodes have happened about annually, but the strange sensation comes at least every two weeks. She was started on phenytoin in her twenties, which she has used sporadically because of dizziness and cognitive problems. After immigrating, she had a tonic-clonic seizure and restarted phenytoin at a dose of 100 mg bid. The primary care physician has also done a routine health checkup and discovered high cholesterol and intends to start simvastatin. Phenytoin is switched to levetiracetam. The side effects are improved and patient reports stricter adherence. New check of blood lipids reveals better levels, so a statin is never started.

> *Comment: Older ASMs with negative effects on blood lipids, enzymeinducing properties interacting with other medications, and substantial side effects are still common. If the epilepsy situation is excellent, there may not be a need to revise the therapy. In this case, where the patient had recent seizures and side effects causing problems with adherence, there was little downside to switching to an ASM with a more favorable profile. As a bonus, the patient would have had better effect of simvastatin, had it been needed to be started (but the lipid profile normalized—it could have been the result of phenytoin). Lamotrigine or lacosamide could have been other options. Carbamazepine and oxcarbazepine are similar in mode of action as phenytoin, and therefore perhaps more likely to cause similar side effects.*

1.10 STATUS EPILEPTICUS

Another advantage of the modern possibilities of compiling and studying large datasets is that it has become possible to study status epilepticus (SE) stratified by etiology. Clearly, the cause of status epilepticus has prognostic implications. Interestingly, remote and acute symptomatic status epilepticus constitute the majority of status epilepticus cases in many large series[31]—which highlights the importance of familiarity with epilepsy in other brain diseases in a wide range of clinical specialties. Globally, status epilepticus seems to differ in presentation and etiology across continents. Convulsive status epilepticus and status epilepticus caused by infections were more commonly encountered in Asia than in Europe and the US, according to a global survey.[32] Access to EEG for diagnosis of non-convulsive cases may account for some of the difference, and a caveat in the interpretation is that determining the incidence of status epilepticus is exceedingly difficult, also with careful ascertainment. Patients may, for instance, die before they present to hospital, and acute symptomatic status epilepticus may only be registered in administrative data as a case of the culprit brain lesion. Recent systematic reviews have shed some light on these difficulties, but the proportion of status epilepticus with remote etiology still varies considerably in the published literature.[33]

Current research on acute symptomatic status epilepticus has also led to new insights on pathophysiological aspects of acquired epilepsy. If an acute symptomatic seizure appears in the form of status epilepticus, the risk of later epilepsy is substantially increased—indicating that either individual vulnerability, SE-induced mechanisms, or lesion characteristics can rapidly accelerate epileptogenesis to a near instant occurrence.[34,35] In fact, some patients seem to have a seizure recurrence risk that is similar to that in epilepsy (but they do not fulfill diagnostic criteria since they have not had an unprovoked seizure). Another relatively recent finding is that the risk of status epilepticus is increased in persons with more than one other brain disease, for instance stroke and dementia.[36] Such studies may inform risk assessment and allow better discussions with patients before considering tapering of ASMs after status epilepticus.

1.11 NON-ASM TREATMENT: POSSIBLE UNDERUTILIZATION

Epilepsy surgery and anti-inflammatory treatment are two potentially disease-modifying treatments that are probably not used enough in patients with epilepsy in other brain diseases. Regarding epilepsy surgery, case series report an underrepresentation of postinfectious, poststroke, and post-traumatic cases in the referred population. The likelihood of successful surgery in most etiologies of epilepsy resulting from another brain disease is therefore hard to elucidate, but such cases exist. More referrals for evaluation could be a first step.

A second large area of possible underutilization of treatment modalities is immunotherapy in immune-mediated epilepsy. Identification of patients with mild autoimmune encephalitis that may benefit form immune treatment could be an enormous leap towards disease modification for the epilepsy field. It will fall on epileptologists or psychiatrists, who are likely to see the patients, to be vigilant in detection. A relatively high seizure frequency and associated cognitive or psychiatric symptoms seem to be important clinical clues. With increased diagnostic suspicion in the absence of good biomarkers, however, there will be a risk of overdiagnosing immune-mediated causes of epilepsy.

1.12 PROGNOSIS: SEIZURES, MORTALITY, AND COMORBIDITIES

The prognosis for persons with epilepsy in other brain diseases is highly variable, as can be expected from the heterogeneous etiologies. Nonetheless, some commonalities emerge across the following chapters. In general, persons with epilepsy after a brain disease report worse quality of life than persons with the same disease that have not developed epilepsy. This is hardly surprising but nonetheless an important point in raising ambitions in management of epilepsy in other brain diseases. Survival is also generally poorer than if epilepsy had not ensued. In most cases, it seems that epilepsy signifies a more serious underlying brain disease: the clearest example is stroke. Patients with poststroke epilepsy survive shorter than patients that have suffered a similar stroke but not developed epilepsy, but not because of seizures; the causes of death are mainly vascular. Similarly, epilepsy-related causes of death are rare in epilepsy after dementia and multiple sclerosis. Instead, epilepsy seems to indicate a severe underlying brain disease. Physicians treating epilepsy should strive not to interfere with treatment of other conditions by choosing antiseizure medications with many interactions. A holistic approach to the patient also involves recognition of all comorbidities and efforts to reduce the risk of for instance vascular events.

That epilepsy-related causes of death are relatively rare compared to other causes does not mean they should be overlooked. Tonic-clonic seizures are potentially lethal and sudden unexpected death in epilepsy (SUDEP) is a matter of great concern also in epilepsy in other brain diseases. Focal epilepsy, structural cause of epilepsy, and particularly post-traumatic epilepsy indicate substantially elevated SUDEP risks in the epilepsy population.[37,38] International guidelines exist about SUDEP information, and it is important that patients with epilepsy in other brain disease and their family are informed in the same manner as in other persons with epilepsy.

1.13 PATIENT-CENTERED OUTCOMES

With an increased focus on epilepsy in other brain disorders, there is also a need for increased research interest in patient-centered outcomes, like quality of life. More work is needed on what patients and caregivers find are the relevant impacts of epilepsy in other brain diseases. In general, patients with epilepsy and another brain disease seem to report worse quality of life than patients who have the same brain disease but do not have epilepsy. The traditional factors associated with low quality of life—seizure freedom, side effects, and psychiatric comorbidity—seem to matter most. This underlines the importance of providing high-quality epilepsy care also if there is another brain disease present. More knowledge, including such that can be obtained from qualitative studies, is needed. Important questions include successful coping mechanisms and obstacles in access to epilepsy care, for instance those related to socioeconomic

TABLE 1.3 Clinical Take-Home Messages

- With ageing populations, epilepsy in other brain diseases—particularly after stroke—becomes more common.
- Epileptogenesis has similarities across brain diseases.
- Avoiding misdiagnosis is important; a first seizure is not always epilepsy in persons with preexisting brain disease.
- Management needs to be as ambitious as for other epilepsies, with tailored ASM selection, follow-up, and therapy revision if needed.

position. Chronic neurological disorders or sequelae from traumatic brain injury or stroke carries obvious risks of a more strained financial situation and other barriers to care, sometimes more so than in cases of idiopathic epilepsy.

There are also health systems challenges. Dissemination of knowledge on particular management aspects of epilepsies caused by different brain disorders needs to improve. With ageing populations, epilepsy after stroke will be a very common epilepsy worldwide, thereby increasing the importance of selecting ASMs that do not have detrimental effects on lipids or interact with stroke prophylaxis. This means that newer ASMs with favorable properties need to be made available. Conversely, increased global mobility makes infectious epilepsies more common everywhere. Clinicians in countries without culprit pathogens will also need to think about infectious causes of epilepsy. Unfortunately, dementias are also increasing in prevalence in many areas of the world. It remains to be seen if more epilepsy in dementia will follow, but barring the unlikely emergence of extremely effective and affordable treatments for Alzheimer's disease, such a development seems likely. The World Health Organization has a global action plan to reduce the impact of epilepsy worldwide. Improved management of epilepsy in other brain diseases will be a very important aspect of that work (Table 1.3).

REFERENCES

1. Adelow C, Andell E, Amark P, Andersson T, Hellebro E, Ahlbom A, et al. Newly diagnosed single unprovoked seizures and epilepsy in Stockholm, Sweden: first report from the Stockholm Incidence Registry of Epilepsy (SIRE). Epilepsia. 2009 May;50:1094–1101.
2. Collaborators GBDE. Global, regional, and national burden of epilepsy, 1990 –2016: a systematic analysis for the Global Burden of Disease Study 2016. Lancet Neurol. 2019 April;18:357–375.
3. Jungehulsing GJ, Heuschmann PU, Holtkamp M, Schwab S, Kolominsky-Rabas PL. Incidence and predictors of post-stroke epilepsy. Acta Neurol. Scand. 2013 June;127:427–430.
4. Westman G, Zelano J. Epilepsy diagnosis after Covid-19: a population-wide study. Seizure. 2022 October;101:11–14.
5. Graham NS, Crichton S, Koutroumanidis M, Wolfe CD, Rudd AG. Incidence and associations of poststroke epilepsy: the prospective South London Stroke Register. Stroke J. Cereb. Circ. 2013 March;44:605–611.

6. Hauser WA, Annegers JF, Rocca WA. Descriptive epidemiology of epilepsy: contributions of population-based studies from Rochester, Minnesota. Mayo Clin. Proc. 1996 June;71:576–586.
7. Scheffer IE, Berkovic S, Capovilla G, Connolly MB, French J, Guilhoto L, et al. ILAE classification of the epilepsies: position paper of the ILAE Commission for Classification and Terminology. Epilepsia. 2017 April;58:512–521.
8. Zelano J, Redfors P, Asberg S, Kumlien E. Association between poststroke epilepsy and death: a nationwide cohort study. Eur. Stroke J. 2016 December;1:272–278. Original research article.
9. Karlander M, Ljungqvist J, Zelano J. Post-traumatic epilepsy in adults: a nationwide register-based study. J. Neurol. Neurosurg. Psychiatry. 2021 March 9;92:617–621.
10. Zelano J, Brigo F, Garcia-Patek S. Increased risk of epilepsy in patients registered in the Swedish Dementia Registry. Eur. J. Neurol. 2020 January;27:129–135.
11. Zelano J, Westman G. Epilepsy after brain infection in adults: a register-based population-wide study. Neurology. 2020 December 15;95:e3213–e3220.
12. Burman J, Zelano J. Epilepsy in multiple sclerosis: a nationwide population-based register study. Neurology. 2017 December 12;89:2462–2468.
13. Beghi E, Giussani G, Costa C, DiFrancesco JC, Dhakar M, Leppik I, et al. The epidemiology of epilepsy in older adults: a narrative review by the ILAE Task Force on Epilepsy in the Elderly. Epilepsia. 2023 March;64:586–601.
14. Syvertsen M, Nakken KO, Edland A, Hansen G, Hellum MK, Koht J. Prevalence and etiology of epilepsy in a Norwegian county: a population based study. Epilepsia. 2015 May;56:699–706.
15. Dagiasi I, Vall V, Kumlien E, Burman J, Zelano J. Treatment of epilepsy in multiple sclerosis. Seizure. 2018 May;58:47–51.
16. Redfors P, Holmegaard L, Pedersen A, Jern C, Malmgren K. Long-term follow-up of post-stroke epilepsy after ischemic stroke: room for improved epilepsy treatment. Seizure. 2020 January 21;76:50–55.
17. Frederiksen KS, Cooper C, Frisoni GB, Frolich L, Georges J, Kramberger MG, et al. A European Academy of Neurology guideline on medical management issues in dementia. Eur. J. Neurol. 2020 October;27:1805–1820.
18. Avila EK, Tobochnik S, Inati SK, Koekkoek JAF, McKhann GM, Riviello JJ, et al. Brain tumor-related epilepsy management: a society for neuro-oncology (SNO) consensus review on current management. Neurol. Oncol. 2024 January 5;26:7–24.
19. Loscher W, Klein P. The pharmacology and clinical efficacy of antiseizure medications: from bromide salts to cenobamate and beyond. CNS Drugs. 2021 September;35:935–963.
20. Perucca P, Scheffer IE. Genetic contributions to acquired epilepsies epilepsy currents. Am. Epilepsy Soc. 2021 January–February;21:5–13.
21. Fisher RS, Acevedo C, Arzimanoglou A, Bogacz A, Cross JH, Elger CE, et al. ILAE official report: a practical clinical definition of epilepsy. Epilepsia. 2014 April;55:475–482.
22. Hesdorffer DC, Benn EK, Cascino GD, Hauser WA. Is a first acute symptomatic seizure epilepsy? Mortality and risk for recurrent seizure. Epilepsia. 2009 May;50:1102–1108.
23. Krumholz A, Wiebe S, Gronseth GS, Gloss DS, Sanchez AM, Kabir AA, et al. Evidence-based guideline: management of an unprovoked first seizure in adults: report of the Guideline Development Subcommittee of the American Academy of Neurology and the American Epilepsy Society. Neurology. 2015 April 21;84:1705–1713.
24. Oto MM. The misdiagnosis of epilepsy: appraising risks and managing uncertainty Seizure. 2017 January;44:143–146.
25. Maloney EM, Chaila E, O'Reilly EJ, Costello DJ. Application of recent international epidemiological guidelines to a prospective study of the incidence of first seizures, newly-diagnosed epilepsy and seizure mimics in a defined geographic region in Ireland. Neuroepidemiology. 2019;53:225–236.

26. Lawn N, Chan J, Lee J, Dunne J. Is the first seizure epilepsy —and when? Epilepsia. 2015 September;56:1425–1431.
27. Misra S, Khan EI, Lam TT, Mazumder R, Gururangan K, Hickman LB, et al. Common pathways of epileptogenesis in patients with epilepsy post-brain injury: findings from a systematic review and meta-analysis. Neurology. 2023 November 27;101:e2243–e2256.
28. Consoli D, Bosco D, Postorino P, Galati F, Plastino M, Perticoni GF, et al. Levetiracetam versus carbamazepine in patients with late poststroke seizures: a multicenter prospective randomized open-label study (EpIC project). Cerebrovasc. Dis. 2012;34:282–289.
29. Marson A, Burnside G, Appleton R, Smith D, Leach JP, Sills G, et al. The SANAD II study of the effectiveness and cost-effectiveness of levetiracetam, zonisamide, or lamotrigine for newly diagnosed focal epilepsy: an open-label, non-inferiority, multicentre, phase 4, randomised controlled trial. Lancet. 2021 April 10;397:1363–1374.
30. Marson AG, Al-Kharusi AM, Alwaidh M, Appleton R, Baker GA, Chadwick DW, et al. The SANAD study of effectiveness of carbamazepine, gabapentin, lamotrigine, oxcarbazepine, or topiramate for treatment of partial epilepsy: an unblinded randomised controlled trial. Lancet. 2007 March 24;369:1000–1015.
31. Kellinghaus C, Rossetti AO, Trinka E, Lang N, May TW, Unterberger I, et al. Factors predicting cessation of status epilepticus in clinical practice: data from a prospective observational registry (SENSE). Ann. Neurol. 2019 March;85:421–432.
32. Ferlisi M, Hocker S, Trinka E, Shorvon S; International Steering Committee of the StEp A. Etiologies and characteristics of refractory status epilepticus cases in different areas of the world: results from a global audit. Epilepsia. 2018 October;59 Suppl 2:100–107.
33. Leitinger M, Trinka E, Zimmermann G, Granbichler CA, Kobulashvili T, Siebert U. Epidemiology of status epilepticus in adults: apples, pears, and oranges—a critical review. Epilepsy Behav. 2020 February;103:106720.
34. Galovic M, Dohler N, Erdelyi-Canavese B, Felbecker A, Siebel P, Conrad J, et al. Prediction of late seizures after ischaemic stroke with a novel prognostic model (the SeLECT score): a multivariable prediction model development and validation study Lancet Neurol. 2018 February;17: 143 –152.
35. Hesdorffer DC, Logroscino G, Cascino G, Annegers JF, Hauser WA. Risk of unprovoked seizure after acute symptomatic seizure: effect of status epilepticus. Ann. Neurol. 1998 December;44:908–912.
36. Bjellvi J, Idegard A, Zelano J. Risk factors for status epilepticus after brain disorders in adults: a multi-cohort national register study. Epilepsy Behav. 2024 July;156:109840.
37. Sveinsson O, Andersson T, Carlsson S, Tomson T. Type, etiology, and duration of epilepsy as risk factors for SUDEP: further analyses of a population-based case-control study. Neurology. 2023 November 27;101:e2257–e2265.
38. Harden C, Tomson T, Gloss D, Buchhalter J, Cross JH, Donner E, et al. Practice guideline summary: sudden unexpected death in epilepsy incidence rates and risk factors: report of the Guideline Development, Dissemination, and Implementation Subcommittee of the American Academy of Neurology and the American Epilepsy Society. Neurology. 2017 April 25;88:1674–1680.

Epilepsy after Stroke and Other Vascular Events

2

2.1 RISK OF EPILEPSY

2.1.1 Prevalence

Cerebrovascular disease is one of the most common causes of epilepsy and by far the most common identifiable cause of epilepsy in developed countries. In Europe, stroke causes about 20% of epilepsy.[1] A recent Norwegian cross-sectional population-based study found a cerebrovascular etiology for 21% of all prevalent epilepsy.[2] Prevalence is sensitive to many factors, including survival of patients with stroke, but the figure gives a rough estimate and clearly illustrates that stroke is one of the most common epilepsy etiologies. It is possible that the prevalence of poststroke epilepsy (PSE) will rise in the following years in countries with older populations and improved acute stroke outcomes.

2.1.2 Incidence

The absolute risk of epilepsy after stroke varies from 3% to over 11%, depending on study method and inclusion criteria. There are estimates on both the lower and the higher end of this spectrum; in a Norwegian population-based study only 2.5% developed epilepsy after ischemic stroke.[3] Similarly, in a Danish longitudinal study, 1197 consecutive patients with stroke were followed for seven years and poststroke epilepsy was detected in 3.2%.[4] A multicenter prospective study on 1897 patients reported late unprovoked seizures (after more than two weeks, a common definition at the time) in 3.8% of patients with brain infarction, out of which 55% developed recurrent seizures.[5] Other investigators report higher incidence, 5% of 1832 prospectively followed patients with ischemic stroke developed poststroke epilepsy after 2.5 years in another study,[6] and the Oxfordshire community stroke project reported a cumulative 11.5% risk of seizures over the first five

DOI: 10.1201/9781003501404-2

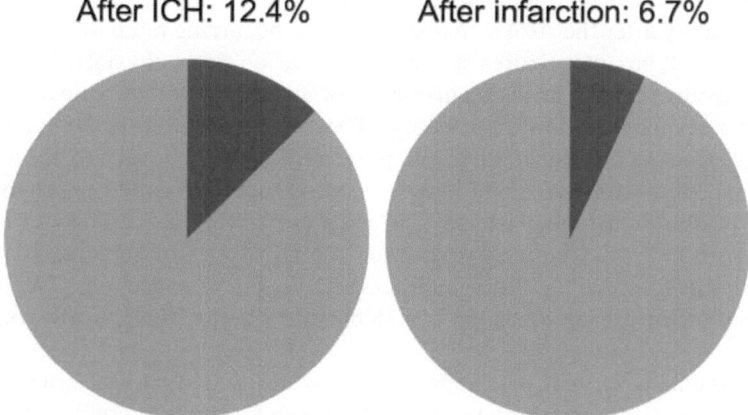

After ICH: 12.4%   After infarction: 6.7%

FIGURE 2.1   Proportion of patients developing epilepsy after stroke in Sweden 2005–2010.[10]

years, but the study did not discriminate between early and late seizures.[7] In a smaller but population-wide study 4.4% of 481 patients developed late seizures over an average follow-up period of 6.3 years.[8] Another study on 1020 patients reported a two-year risk of 8.2%.[9] In 2016 a population-wide study using administrative data from comprehensive registers in Sweden found that approximately 6% of patients developed epilepsy after an ischemic stroke and 12% after hemorrhagic stroke (Figure 2.1), and the later finding was replicated in Finland the year after.[10,11] Studies based in tertiary stroke centers tend to find higher rates, presumably because of more severe strokes. Overall, the variations in incidence is likely to reflect differences in methodology and study populations, perhaps because of differences in which patients have been treated for stroke.

Because of the overall survival after stroke, survival-adjusted risks of epilepsy are higher than absolute risks. In one of the larger studies to date, which followed 3310 patients with newly diagnosed stroke in the UK for an average of 3.8 years, the 10-year survival-adjusted risk of PSE was calculated to be 12.4%.[12] Most patients that develop poststroke epilepsy have their first unprovoked seizure within two years after the first stroke,[6] with a median of about one year.[10–12]

2.2 EPILEPTOGENESIS

Clues about epileptogenesis after stroke can be derived from animal models as well as clinical observations, and there is an ongoing discussion on how well animal models translate to the human condition. In mice and rats, photothrombotic stroke or internal carotid ligature are models of ischemic stroke, and different forms of intracerebral hemorrhage (ICH) can be used to model poststroke epilepsy and tend to show inflammation and network remodeling during epileptogenesis.[13]

In humans there is an important distinction between early seizures, which occur at or immediately after the stroke, and late seizures occurring more than a week after stroke.[14] These types of seizures are presumed to be pathophysiologically different. Early seizures have a lower recurrence risk and are therefore believed to reflect an acute but reversible brain disturbance. They are considered acute symptomatic and do not necessarily reflect that epileptogenesis has occurred. To the contrary, late seizures occur after the acute injury. Such seizures are called unprovoked and have a very high recurrence risk, in fact often motivating a diagnosis of epilepsy. Importantly, a too strict boundary between the two types of seizures is probably an oversimplification from a biological perspective. For instance, early seizures are a major risk factor for late ones, so it is debatable whether there is always a latent period.[15]

Most patients have their first unprovoked seizure in the first year after stroke, so epileptogenic mechanisms are likely to involve tissue reactions operating on that temporal scale; network reorganization and postinjury brain responses like inflammation and glia scarring. In animal models as well as humans, lesion characteristics are the most important determinants of the risk of poststroke epilepsy, and extensive brain damage involving the cortex is most likely to cause epilepsy.[15,16] The inflammatory response to the stroke, including both the acute response and later glial scarring, seems to influence the likelihood of epilepsy.[13]

There is emerging evidence suggesting that a more rapid epileptogenesis indicates a more aggressive poststroke epilepsy.[17,18] Acute symptomatic seizures at the onset of stroke are a strong risk factor for subsequent epilepsy, and particularly so if the acute symptomatic seizure is a status epilepticus.[17,19] Whether the association between acute symptomatic seizures and later poststroke epilepsy represents an unfortunate network disruption that immediately gives rise to epilepsy, that patients with acute symptomatic seizures have individual susceptibility with regards to preexisting seizure threshold, or if the acute symptomatic seizure itself is epileptogenic is not known. Some evidence exists to support at least the two first explanations, which may well apply in different patients. A role for strategic network disruption is supported by the fact that stroke in different bran regions infers different risks of poststroke epilepsy.[20] Individual susceptibility is supported by epidemiologic and imaging studies showing that vascular disease and cerebrovascular small vessel disease increase the risk of epilepsy.[21,22] Longitudinal studies repeatedly show that vascular risk factors like hypertension increases the risk of epilepsy in later life. Imaging studies further support a role for microvascular lesions. Indirect measures of glymphatic system components like enlarged periventricular spaces are also possible risk factors for poststroke epilepsy.[22,23]

Genetic vulnerability does not seem to play a major role but cannot be completely discarded as one contributor to epileptogenesis after stroke. The relative risk of poststroke epilepsy is 20% higher in persons with a first-degree relative with epilepsy.[24] Although this is significant, the small magnitude of the risk means that stroke characteristics like size, location, and hemorrhage by far outweigh any genetic contribution. Some small studies have found gene variants associated with increased epilepsy risk.[25,26]

There have been several attempts to stop epileptogenesis after stroke. In animals, drugs like statins, antiseizure medications, and inflammation modulators can reduce the risk of experimentally induced epilepsy.[27–31] In humans, promising results have been scarce (Table 2.1).

Trials trying to find actual antiepileptogenesis effects of ASMs have so far been negative. Observational studies indicate that treatment with statins might reduce the risk of PSE, particularly in patients with acute symptomatic seizures.[6,32] These are a high-risk group for poststroke epilepsy, so it is possible that this enrichment of a high-risk population was necessary to find a true antiepilepsy effect. Whether this is due to an actual antiepileptic effect or reduction of risk for subsequent vascular events is not known.

2.2.1 Stroke Treatment to Prevent Epileptogenesis

The most direct way to prevent epilepsy after stroke would be to prevent or mitigate the initial stroke. Early studies on revascularization therapies were very small, for instance one investigation on 257 patients treated with IV thrombolysis reported a rate of late epileptic seizures of 11.3%.[33] The figure is very similar to another study that retrospectively compared cases that had received t-PA with controls that had not and found no significant difference in epilepsy incidence at two years (10.8% for t-PA vs 8.0% for controls).[34] Lately, larger studies including thrombectomy seem to have clarified the matter. In a study based on the Swedish stroke register, investigators studied all patients that had undergone thrombectomy for acute ischemic stroke.[35] Poststroke epilepsy developed in 7.9%, but the risk was 6.5% (95% CI = 5.28%–7.70%) after thrombectomy,

TABLE 2.1   Examples of Studies Trying to Prevent Epileptogenesis or Early Seizures

ANTIEPILEPTOGENESIS/EARLY SEIZURES	
RANDOMIZED TRIALS	
STUDY	RESULT
Gilad et al. 2011[36]	Valproate for one month did not result in fewer patients with late seizures after ICH compared to placebo. Fewer patients with early seizures in VPA group (nonsignificant difference).
Peter-Derex et al. 2022[37]	Levetiracetam resulted in fewer acute symptomatic seizures compared to placebo in first 72 h after ICH.
OBSERVATIONAL STUDIES	
Zhu et al. 2022[38]	Fewer cases of poststroke epilepsy in double dose compared to standard dose statin in patients with ischemic stroke.
Guo et al. 2015[6]	Fewer early seizures and fewer cases of poststroke epilepsy in patients with early seizures in statin users.
Passero et al. 2002[39]	Fewer early seizures in patients using ASMs after ICH.

compared to 10.0% (95% CI = 8.25%–11.75%) after thrombolysis, and 12.3% after no revascularization (95% CI = 10.33%–14.25%). All groups were matched on admission stroke severity, so it seems that mitigating the stroke also reduces the risk of poststroke epilepsy. Predictors of epilepsy after thrombectomy were large infarction on imaging after treatment, high posttreatment NIHSS, and need of assistance three months after stroke—all indicators of a severe stroke despite treatment.[35] Recently, Danish researchers reported similar findings.[40]

2.2.2 Biomarkers

Animal work and the clear role of stroke characteristics in determining epilepsy risk has led to a great interest in biomarkers that can predict epilepsy after stroke or indicate that epileptogenesis is taking place. So far, there are no robust markers useful for clinical practice. Proteomics in blood at the acute stroke shows that patients that later develop epilepsy have lower S100B and Hsc70, and upregulated endostatin.[41] Other markers like the cell adhesion molecule NCAM was higher in patients with acute stroke that had early seizures, whereas TNF-alpha was lower.[42] Traditional brain injury markers like neurofilament are high in patients with stroke that later develop epilepsy, but this is hardly surprising given that severe stroke is a risk factor and the added value of biochemical markers is uncertain.[43] Once epilepsy has developed, patients with poststroke epilepsy exhibit higher blood levels of neurofilament and S100B than persons without epilepsy, but again the value of these proteins as clinical markers is uncertain.[44]

Imaging biomarkers have mainly been used to quantify stroke volume, which is a predictor of poststroke epilepsy. Similarly, cortical involvement is a risk factor, whereas subcortical location does not seem to increase the risk of poststroke epilepsy.[45]

EEG is another readily available biomarker that is perhaps not used to its full potential. It is clear that with longer monitoring of patients with acute stroke, yield with regards to epileptiform activity will increase.[45] For instance, a recent study using 48-hour EEG monitoring detected acute symptomatic electrographic seizures in nearly half of ICH patients that did not receive antiseizure medication.[33] Another study of severe ischemic stroke found electrographic acute symptomatic seizures in 26% and most were electrographic only.[46] Some studies have found that early epileptiform activity predicts later poststroke epilepsy, which is not very surprising given that, clinically, early seizures are a risk factor for later ones. Perhaps in the future, EEG monitoring will allow better monitoring of patients at high risk of poststroke epilepsy.

2.2.2.1 Pre-Stroke Seizures

Pre-stroke seizures refer to new-onset seizures in a person of middle age or above who shortly thereafter suffers stroke, the clinical perception being that the seizure has heralded a stroke. The phenomenon has been reported in the literature for decades, but only recently with regards to management implications. In the Oxfordshire community study, 19 (3%) of 675 patients with subsequent stroke had previous seizures and seven patients had a first seizure in the year before their stroke.[7] In a case-control study on

230 patients with stroke, 4.5% of patients had previous epilepsy compared to 0.6% of controls.[47] These observations were recently confirmed and quantified in population-wide register studies.[48,49] After middle age, a first seizure carries a nearly two-fold relative risk of subsequent stroke.[49] The risk is similarly increased in women and men, but seems to diminish in the very old. In absolute terms, a first seizure in middle age can be expected to be followed by stroke in 5%–20% of patients within 10 years.[48]

Pre-stroke seizures are an additional example of the close link between vascular health and late-onset seizures, and evidence is accumulating that late-onset epilepsy is often associated with high vascular risk. For instance, midlife vascular risk factors increase the risk of late-onset epilepsy.[21] The phenomenon of pre-stroke seizures illustrates the reverse: seizures revealing vascular lesion burden. It seems likely that screening patients with new-onset seizures after middle age for vascular risk factors and intervention as directed by local guidelines would be beneficial, but firm evidence about the value of such a policy is lacking. Such interventions could probably include smoking cessations and blood pressure management. Other than clinical judgment, there have been no studies investigating whether late-onset seizures should be treated as TIA equivalents. The risk of stroke after a first seizure seems lower than that after TIA, but still substantial. More research is needed.

CASE 2.1 Pre-Stroke Seizures

A 69-year-old female is referred for a first unprovoked tonic-clonic seizure. An ER CT is unremarkable, and she is seen in the first seizure clinic where she denies any previous paroxysmal symptoms. An MRI performed six weeks after the first seizure shows a small subacute left frontoparietal subcortical infarction, according to the radiology report no more than two weeks old. At the follow-up visit, the patient and her husband describe an episode of right arm apraxia and impressive dysphasia that resolved spontaneously after five minutes, about a week before the MRI.

Comment: The case illustrates the concept of pre-stroke seizures. The MRI infarction happened after the first seizure and reflects the symptoms that occurred about a month after the first seizure.

2.3 RISK FACTORS

Clinical risk factors that increase the risk of poststroke epilepsy are mainly related to stroke characteristics. Severe stroke, stroke affecting the cortex, and bleeding carry the greatest risk. Surrogate markers of large and often cortical stroke like atrial fibrillation are also associated with increased risk of poststroke epilepsy. Acute symptomatic seizures are another important risk factor. Young age seems to increase the risk slightly.[10–12,50]

TABLE 2.2   Risk Factors for Poststroke Epilepsy According to the CAVE and Select Models

MODEL	CAVE[51]	SELECT[50]
STROKE TYPE	ICH	ISCHEMIC STROKE

Risk factors	cortical involvement
	age <65 years
	volume >10 mL
	early seizures
		NIHSS
		Large-artery atherosclerosis
		Short acute symptomatic
		  seizure
		Acute symptomatic status
		  epilepticus
		Cortical involvement
		Territory of middle cerebral
		  artery

Risk of poststroke epilepsy if highest score	46%	100%

There are several risk scores that try to predict poststroke epilepsy, among the more well-known ones are SELECT and CAVE (Table 2.2). The SELECT score is a nine-point scale in which the highest score carries a >80% (95% CI 62%–93%) risk of poststroke epilepsy. The model is named after the most important risk factors: severity of stroke, large-artery atherosclerotic etiology, early seizures, cortical involvement, and territory of middle cerebral artery involvement, and can be calculated manually or through a smartphone app.[50] The CAVE score is a corresponding scale for hemorrhagic stroke.[51] So far, these scores and others do not have major clear management implications, but they may be used to tailor patient information and vigilance for seizures in those particularly at-risk.

2.4 RISK AFTER THE FIRST SEIZURE

2.4.1 Risk of Epilepsy after an Acute Symptomatic Seizure

Acute symptomatic (early) seizures occur within the first week after stroke. The frequency of early seizures after stroke varies greatly between studies, probably for methodological reasons like variation in stroke severity between populations. The risk factors for early seizures parallel those of poststroke epilepsy: hemorrhage and cortical involvement are the most prominent ones.[52–54] The risk of subsequent epilepsy after an early seizure is about 30%.[55,56] A more precise estimate can sometimes be obtained using the aforementioned SELECT or CAVE scores.[50,51]

Clinically, the risk estimate conveyed to the patient with an acute symptomatic seizure should be at least approximately that of a first unprovoked seizure without a brain lesion. It is important to recognize and convey to the patient that the risk of epilepsy is not negligible; we now know that a significant proportion of patients will develop epilepsy.

CASE 2.2 Acute Symptomatic Seizure

A 68-year-old female has a right parietal lobe cortical stroke with hemorrhagic transformation and has an acute symptomatic seizure while in hospital. She is started on levetiracetam, which is withdrawn after three months. Three weeks later she has two focal to bilateral tonic-clonic seizures, is diagnosed with poststroke epilepsy and restarted on ASM therapy.

>   *Comment: Given that the patient had only had an acute symptomatic seizure, it was not unreasonable to taper the ASM. The important thing is to inform the patient that the acute symptomatic seizure indicates a risk of epilepsy and involvement in the course of action.*

2.4.2 Risk of Epilepsy after an Unprovoked Poststroke Seizure

Unprovoked seizures are seizures occurring more than seven days after the stroke. Such seizures carry a substantial recurrence risk of nearly 70%.[56] The ILAE definition of epilepsy allows epilepsy diagnosis already after a first unprovoked seizures after stroke, because the recurrence risk is similar to with that seen after two unprovoked seizures in any individual.[57] It is important to note that the study upon which the ILAE based its definition is from an era with less advanced imaging than today.[58] The high recurrence risks may for instance not extend to all patients with small or lacunar stroke detected on MRI.

Importantly, a first seizure more than two years after stroke seem to have a lower risk[18]—presumably because a greater proportion of seizures occurring at that time interval are unrelated to the stroke. In a Swedish case series the median latency to the first late seizure was 283 days (55 days in the earliest case).[59]

2.4.3 Risk after Other Stroke Forms/ Hypoperfusion Injuries

Ischemic and hemorrhagic stroke are the most common stroke forms and dominate the literature. Epilepsy can also arise from other vascular causes, including subarachnoid hemorrhage, cerebral sinuous venous thrombosis, and hypoxic-ischemic encephalopathy after cardiac arrest.

2.4.3.1 Subarachnoid Hemorrhage

Subarachnoid hemorrhage is relatively more common in young stroke patients. It is rare compared to other stroke subtypes, and so it accounts for a small proportion of all cases of poststroke epilepsy but seems to carry a substantial risk, at least comparable to that after ICH.[7,12,60,61] The five-year risk of epilepsy is probably approximately 12%. Risk factors include bleeding size, and the median time to epilepsy was eight months in one study.[60,62] Reported frequencies of acute symptomatic seizures vary but are relatively similar to those seen after ICH.

2.4.3.2 Central Venous Sinus Thrombosis

Cerebral venous sinuous thrombosis can cause venous congestion infarctions in turn causing seizures. In a large multicenter study, acute symptomatic seizures occurred in 34%.[63] The risk factors were ICH, cerebral edema/infarction without ICH, cortical vein thrombosis, superior sagittal sinus thrombosis, focal neurologic deficit, sulcal subarachnoid hemorrhage, and female sex. Importantly, many cases of cerebral venous thrombosis are detected because of seizures, and only 7% of the cohort ($n = 1281$) had postdiagnosis acute symptomatic seizures only. Status epilepticus in the acute symptomatic phase occurred in 6%. Risk factors of SE was ICH, focal neurologic deficits, and cerebral edema/infarction. Acute symptomatic seizures were not independently associated with outcome.

Unprovoked seizures, occurring more than seven days after diagnosis of cerebral venous thrombosis, were also studied in the same cohort.[64] Eleven percent developed unprovoked seizures. Risk factors were acute symptomatic seizures, neurosurgery, subdural hematoma, and ICH. The median time to epilepsy was five months. Interestingly, 70% of the 123 patients with one unprovoked seizure had a seizure recurrence despite ASM therapy. This suggests that a first unprovoked seizure after cerebral venous thrombosis is indicative of epilepsy in the same manner as after other types of stroke.

2.4.3.3 Hypoxic-Ischemic Encephalopathy

Although not stroke, cardiac arrest causes reduction of brain blood supply leading to brain damage that can sometimes cause seizures. Postanoxic convulsions can follow in many different forms. There has been much focus lately on the prognostic implications of status epilepticus after cardiac arrest, which is slightly outside the scope of this book. In short, the issue is whether patients remain unconscious because of epileptic activity in the brain or if such activity is a mere epiphenomenon of the brain injury.[65] In the latter case, ASM treatment would matter less for prognosis.

It is now clear that all postanoxic status epilepticus do not indicate a hopeless prognosis. Almost 25% of some cohorts go on to wake up.[66–68] Survivors typically had preserved brain stem reflexes, preserved N20 responses, and otherwise favorable indicators suggesting that there has been no catastrophic brain injury. Attempts are therefore often made in such cases to treat the electrographic seizure activity with ASMs or propofol while maintaining supporting care. The field is rapidly evolving. A recent randomized trial did not show that standardized treatment with ASMs according to traditional status epilepticus protocols aimed at suppressing seizures in non-hypoxic-ischemic cases improved prognosis.[69] Current guidelines state that EEG should be performed after cardiac arrest, but any prognostication should be based on a multimodal assesment.[70]

Lance–Adam syndrome refers to action/intention myoclonus after cardiac arrest.[71] The term is sometimes applied more widely to all sorts of postanoxic myoclonia. Many different ASMs have been used with varying degrees of success, and the literature is restricted to case series. Myoclonia are sometimes interpreted as a very negative prognostic sign after cardiac arrest, but this is not a good clinical rule.[72] If myoclonia occur against a continuous reactive EEG background, it may be what was called "Lance–Adam precursor" pattern, which does not indicate a poor prognosis.[73]

Survivors of cardiac arrest have only a somewhat increased risk of epilepsy. One large study found a hazard ratio of 1.8 compared to age-matched controls and a cumulative incidence of 1.26% compared to 0.61%.[74] The low risk probably reflects the subcortical nature of the injury type. In 32 survivors of cardiac arrest that underwent outpatient EEG as part of their follow-up, 11 had epilepsy. The clinical presentation varied from tonic-clonic seizures (5) to myoclonus (3) and behavioral arrest (3).[75]

2.5 MANAGEMENT

2.5.1 Clinical Presentation

Seizures at or after stroke are focal onset, but relatively often bilateral tonic-clonic. In one series about 10% of acute symptomatic seizures were focal aware seizures, 25% were focal impaired awareness, and 55% were bilateral tonic-clonic.[76] Most seizures (76%) occurred before arrival to the hospital. Acute symptomatic seizures are also probably underrecognized once patients are admitted; large recent studies using video-EEG in severe acute stroke have revealed that one out of six of patients have clinical or subclinical early seizures.[37] The semiology of seizures later after stroke—when the patient is considered to have epilepsy—is less often bilateral tonic-clonic. One study reported that only 13% were bilateral tonic-clonic, 17% focal impaired awareness, and 67% focal aware seizures.[77] Other investigators have seen somewhat higher rates of bilateral tonic-clonic seizures, but still found that over 40% of poststroke epilepsy seizures were non-motor onset, and the majority of such patients did not have any convulsions.[78] The semiology studies show the need for vigilance for focal seizures in stroke survivors and recognition that motor signs are not always present. The differences between acute symptomatic seizures and later poststroke epilepsy seizures are interesting (Figure 2.2)—tonic-clonic seizures could be more common early after stroke for biological reasons; alternatively the difference may reflect underrecognition of focal seizures in the acute phase (see Epileptogenesis section).

In the clinical examination, decreased consciousness can suggest a focal impaired awareness seizure. Other clues to ongoing seizure activity can be subtle jerking or twitching, nystagmus, or conjugate gaze away from the side of the brain with the seizure focus (towards the motor impaired extremity). Repeated history-taking is sometimes helpful and can reveal convulsions at symptom onset or during transport. A particular challenge is patients with previous stroke that present with new symptoms. They are at risk of both a new stroke and poststroke epilepsy.

2.5.2 Seizures as Stroke Mimics and Chameleons

Acute symptomatic seizures can be a complex clinical challenge. Clinically, it is often not possible to distinguish a postictal paresis after an acute symptomatic seizure caused by stroke from a postictal paresis after a focal seizure unrelated to a stroke. Since revascularization is time sensitive, some unnecessary investigations and even revascularization treatments are probably unavoidable. Clinical judgment and awareness of the potential pitfall is important.

Acute symptomatic seizures occur most often in the first 24–48 hours of stroke, not seldom at stroke onset.[6] In most countries, an acute symptomatic seizure is not a contraindication to revascularization with thrombolysis or thrombectomy if the cause is thought to be ischemic stroke, so clinicians on call are faced with the problems of both stroke mimics (seizures misinterpreted as stroke) and stroke chameleons (seizures caused by a stroke that is overlooked). Most important for avoiding missing a stroke is recognition of the fact that seizures can be acute symptomatic. In the large revascularization trials, about 1.5% of patients treated with IV thrombolysis had a seizure at stroke onset, and this was later considered a mimic (there was no stroke) in about 40%.[76] Observational studies suggest that advanced imaging (CT angiogram and CT perfusion or MRI) can help clinicians identify stroke in need of revascularization in cases where a first seizure is suspected to be acute symptomatic due to stroke.[76,79]

2.5.3 Estimating Recurrence Risk

There are some caveats with simply diagnosing epilepsy after all first seizures in patients with previous stroke (Figure 2.3). First, one needs to be sure that the seizure is not an acute symptomatic seizure caused by a new stroke or other factors. Second, it is often wise to consider the temporal relationship between the previous stroke and the new-onset seizure. Most cases of poststroke epilepsy have an onset within the first year after stroke, and 90% have their first seizure within two years.[6] Since poststroke epilepsy features focal-onset seizures, the semiology can sometimes be related to the stroke location—which strengthens the diagnosis. Seizures with a suspected different anatomical origin or arising more than two years after a stroke should raise suspicions of an alternative cause. Similarly, most studies evaluating risks of poststroke epilepsy only included patients with clinically manifest stroke. It is therefore not clear whether a silent older stroke detected on MRI in a first seizure work-up should be given the same diagnostic weight. The recurrence risk in such cases is currently not known.

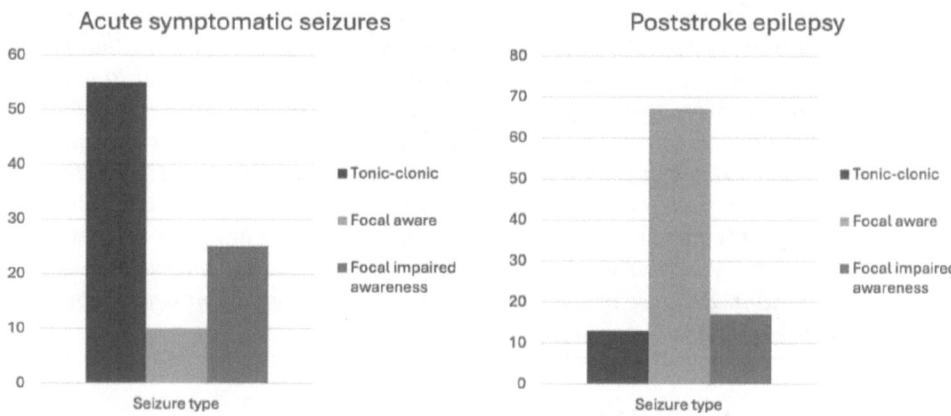

FIGURE 2.2 Reported proportions of clinically overt seizure types in acute symptomatic and late poststroke seizures.[76,77] Whether the difference reflects underrecognition of focal acute symptomatic seizures or biological differences is unclear. Importantly, many poststroke epilepsy seizures are focal and potentially missed.

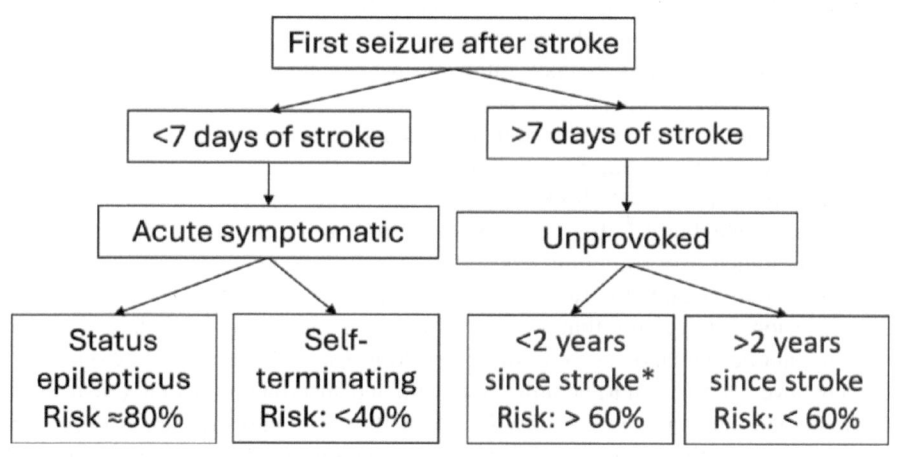

FIGURE 2.3 Risk estimates in different clinical situations.

Note: * Diagnosis of epilepsy can be considered.

CASE 2.3 Unclear Recurrence Risk

A 74-year-old male with hypertension is referred after a first unprovoked seizure, which was a tonic-clonic seizure with unknown onset (the seizure woke his wife while ongoing). His first seizure work-up is a normal routine EEG. MRI reveals a 1 cm large white matter lacunar infarction. He reports never having any stroke symptoms.

Comment: The case illustrates detection of a previous silent stroke in a first seizure work-up. Although the ILAE definition paper[57] indicates that a first seizure after stroke qualifies as epilepsy, it may not extend to this situation. Most if not all data on recurrence risk after stroke is from clinically overt stroke. In addition, subcortical strokes may not indicate increased recurrence risk in the same degree as cortical stroke. Finally, the latency from the stroke to the seizure is unknown. In this case, there is probably not evidence of a recurrence risk motivating an epilepsy diagnosis. Vascular work-up and appropriate risk factor intervention is important. Because of the vascular risk factors, the patient is probably at risk of late-onset epilepsy.

2.5.4 Neurological Worsening after Seizures

A current paradigm in epilepsy is that seizures are a signaling problem not causing brain damage, except for prolonged status epilepticus. Nonetheless, many clinicians will encounter cases of poststroke seizures where neurological function does not seem to recover fully. The phenomenon is often explained as an extended period of postictal paresis, which may sometimes be the case. There are however alternative explanations, including that seizures may indeed cause persisting damage. In Lausanne, Switzerland, about 20% of a series of 48 patients exhibited neurological worsening that was considered persistent, which is not typical for a postictal paresis.[80] In Ghent, Belgium, the median modified Rankin Score (mRS) score in 72 patients with seizures after stroke worsened from a median of 3 to a median of 4 after the seizure.[81] Finally, a study from Rochester, MN, USA, found that in a cohort developing poststroke epilepsy, the mean mRS was 2.9 after the stroke, but 3.3 after development of poststroke epilepsy.[8] The pathophysiology of neurological worsening after poststroke seizures probably varies across patients. In addition to an extended period of a postictal paresis, imaging can sometimes show enlarged lesions, suggesting that already stroke-damaged tissue is perhaps extra sensitive to metabolic demands such as those resulting from a seizure.[81] Alternatively, the area may have been vascularly challenged again and sustained new injury, causing both the seizure and the worsening. An MRI study with scans obtained soon after poststroke seizures illustrated the panorama of causes; some patients had signal changes suggesting cytotoxic edema around the old infarction, whereas others seemed to have had a new stroke (that group had cardioembolic etiology),[82] so it would seem that not all cases of neurological worsening after poststroke seizures are standard postictal paresis.

2.5.5 Treatment of Early Seizures

There is no evidence on how to treat acute symptomatic poststroke seizures. These are often one-time occurrences with a recurrence risk of 10%–20% for more acute symptomatic seizures. Because of the low recurrence risk, some authorities caution against overtreatment with ASMs,[83] which should probably be avoided to prevent unnecessary side effects that may harm rehabilitation. Although ASMs prevent seizures while treatment is ongoing,[37] there is no evidence yet that they prevent subsequent epilepsy. On the other hand, seizure-related risks should recurrence occur can sometimes balance the equation—making treatment the best choice from a risk–benefit perspective. In cases of multiple acute symptomatic seizures, a very unstable cerebrovascular situation where blood pressure control is essential, if the first seizure was prolonged, in the presence of fractures that need to be immobilized, or a multitude of other scenarios, one may want to minimize the risk of seizure recurrence, which may motivate treatment with ASMs after an acute symptomatic seizure. Acute symptomatic status epilepticus needs treatment according to local status epilepticus guidelines. Levetiracetam is a common first choice, but there are other alternatives.

If treatment is initiated to prevent further acute symptomatic seizures, it is helpful to document the treatment objective so that patients are not left on ASMs for long time periods without reflection. Most experts suggest that the duration of treatment should be kept short, but there is no firm evidence and clinical judgment must prevail.[83,84] In some uncomplicated cases, treatment for seven days to cover the acute symptomatic phase can be sufficient. In cases of remaining intracerebral blood, if the first seizure has been particularly severe, or if there are several risk factors for subsequent epilepsy—longer treatment may be warranted. A common practice is to treat for three to six months. Acute symptomatic status epilepticus seems to indicate a very high risk, as discussed later. It is important to involve the patient and caregivers in shared decision-making before any withdrawal.

In the acute symptomatic phase, one needs to select an ASM that can be quickly administered without the need for titration, and ideally has an IV formulation. Levetiracetam is a common choice.[83] Other options include valproic acid, phenytoin, and lacosamide, but the potential for drug–drug interactions argue against the first two and the sodium-blocking mode of action of lacosamide may not be ideal for vascularly ill patients, although the drug is gaining popularity.

Withdrawing an ASM that has been started to prevent acute symptomatic seizure recurrence is generally slow—tapering should take at least a few weeks. If a late seizure occurs it is hopefully mitigated somewhat by the ASM treatment. There is no firm evidence, so the exact time period needs to be decided on a case-by-case basis and with a well-informed patient participating in deciding the appropriate duration.[83] Caution is warranted in cases of acute symptomatic status epilepticus, which greatly increases the risk of subsequent epilepsy—particularly if the stroke is severe.[16,85,86] Large studies using administrative data in the US have shown that convulsive status epilepticus after stroke is associated with a four-fold increased risk of death.[87]

2.5.6 Treatment of Epilepsy

In selecting ASMs for poststroke epilepsy, the most important considerations are side effects and drug–drug interactions. If possible, the epilepsy treatment should not interfere with the carefully tailored stroke secondary prophylaxis. Drug–drug interactions can mainly arise with enzyme-inducing drugs. These are not only theoretical risks; lipid-lowering statins are less effective in older patients treated with carbamazepine than in patients treated with lamotrigine or levetiracatam.[88] Newer generation ASMs with enzyme-inducing properties can also lower the concentrations of simvastatin.[89,90] The combination of strong enzyme inducers, exemplified by carbamazepine and phenytoin, with new anticoagulants like apixaban or dabigatran, is discouraged in the prescription information. Older antiepileptic drugs may be even more harmful than previously appreciated. A study on Swedish prescription data found that use of valproic acid was associated with an increased risk of death, also with adjustment for factors that may have affected ASM choice.[91]

Regarding vascular risk, ASMs can in themselves impact serum lipids, weight, and perhaps the risk of cardiac arythmias.[92] The literature on the effect of ASM *per se* on lipids is not unequivocal. Negative effects seem larger for older-generation ASMs, but this may reflect publication bias or lack of data, as noted in a recent systematic review.[90]

Regarding effect on seizures, some guidance can be drawn from studies on epilepsy in the elderly in general, since stroke is such a common etiology. Levetiracetam was shown to have better tolerability than controlled-release carbamazepine in an elderly population with epilepsy of predominantly cerebrovascular aetiology.[93] Lamotrigine performed closely to levetiracetam in the same study but was not statistically significantly different from levetiracetam or carbamazepine. Several studies have shown that lamotrigine and levetiracetam are well tolerated in older patients with focal epilepsy.[93–95] In the SANAD trial on partial epilepsy,[96] gabapentin seemed slightly less effective than other drugs, but the drug was reported as efficacious in one uncontrolled study in poststroke epilepsy (see next).

2.5.6.1 ASMs Specifically Studied in Poststroke Epilepsy

Levetiracetam has also been evaluated in non-blinded prospective studies on patients with poststroke epilepsy and shown to be tolerated and effective.[97] Lamotrigine and levetiracetam have also outperformed carbamazepine regarding side effects, but not regarding effect on seizures in patients with epilepsy after stroke in two randomized trials.[98,99] In the first, the rate of seizure freedom was modest and the trial included only 64 patients with late poststroke seizures comparing carbamazepine and lamotrigine.[98] Seizure freedom was achieved in 44% and 72%, respectively. The difference in efficacy was not statistically significant, but the difference in withdrawal due to side effects was, with lamotrigine being better tolerated.[98] The other often-cited randomized open-label trial included 128 patients and compared levetiracetam to slow-release carbamazepine. The study demonstrated no significant difference in effect on seizures, but cognitive side effects were less frequent in the levetiracetam group.[99] However, the difference effect size was small: seizure freedom was achieved in 94% of patients treated with levetiracetam and 85% of patients treated with carbamazepine, and the authors note that the study was initially designed for a much larger population.

Most studies on treatment of poststroke epilepsy are small, illustrating the difficulty of including and following patients with symptomatic epilepsy over time (Table 2.3). A meta-analysis confirmed that particularly lamotrigine seems to be a well-tolerated choice.[100] The slow titration required argues against selecting lamotrigine in cases where rapid effect is needed, like seizure clusters or very frequent seizures. In a

TABLE 2.3   Selected Studies on Treatment of Poststroke Epilepsy

RANDOMIZED TRIALS	
STUDY	*RESULT*
Consoli et al. 2012[99]	No difference in proportion achieving seizure freedom with levetiracetam vs carbamazepine. Fewer side effects with levetiracetam.
Gilad et al. 2007[98]	72% seizure free with lamotrigine vs 44% with carbamazepine (but not significant); fewer side effects with lamotrigine.
OBSERVATIONAL STUDIES	
Kutlu et al. 2008[97]	82% seizure free with levetiracetam monotherapy.
Alvarez-Sabin et al. 2002[101]	18% had seizure recurrence with gabapentin monotherapy.

Swedish register-based study, lamotrigine and levetiracetam had higher retention rates than carbamazepine in epilepsy after stroke.[102] A study by Alvarez-Sabin and co-workers studied gabapentin in patients with epilepsy after stroke: in an uncontrolled investigation on 71 patients with a first late seizure, the drug was well tolerated and seizures recurred in only 18.3% during the mean follow up of 30 months.[101]

2.5.7 Withdrawal of ASMs

Currently, there is scarcity of data for information on which patients can withdraw ASMs once poststroke epilepsy has developed. In some cohorts, structural cause, abnormal neurological examination, and onset in adulthood are factors associated with a higher risk of seizure recurrence, indicating that patients with poststroke epilepsy could be a high-risk group.[103] In most cases, ASM withdrawal is not advisable if the patient wants to maximize chances to remain seizure free. Patients need to be counselled carefully before attempting withdrawal to ensure that they fully appreciate the risks of seizure recurrence.

2.6 PROGNOSIS

2.6.1 Seizures

The seizure prognosis in poststroke epilepsy is variable. Older literature usually describes poststroke epilepsy as easy to treat, with monotherapy being sufficient.[8,104] This is probably an oversimplification. It is true that in randomized clinical trials, the remission rates have often been high. However, in retrospective studies—describing

TABLE 2.4 Risk Factors of Pharmacoresistance

Severe stroke
Bleeding/ICH
Short latency to first seizure
Status epilepticus

the actual real-world outcome—seizure freedom rates are much lower.[59,105] In a Swedish retrospective series we found that 46% became seizure free on their first ASM, and 55% on the second or third.[59] There are several possible interpretations. If the clinical trials represent the general patient population, one could argue that poststroke epilepsy is biologically easy to treat. This raises the issue whether physicians are perhaps not ambitious enough in our pursuit of seizure freedom in poststroke patients. Another possibility is that the clinical trials have been subject to selection bias and that the retrospective studies better represent patients encountered in clinical care. It is possible that patients with very severe stroke and poststroke epilepsy were not included.

Pharmacoresistance occurs in at least 20% of cases, and in some series at least one third requires more than one ASM.[17,106] One study of more than 150 patients found that factors predicting pharmacoresistance included those associated with risk of poststroke epilepsy in general, like ICH and large stroke. Interestingly, latency and status epilepticus were in addition to the traditional factors significant contributor to the risk of pharmacoresistance. In fact, if epilepsy developed within the first six months after stroke, the risk of pharmacoresistance was nearly one hundred times higher than if epilepsy developed more than a year after stroke, and status epilepticus increased the risk with a factor of 14.[17] Clinically, this means that patients with short latency to their epilepsy may merit particular monitoring and follow-up with regards to pharmacoresistance (Table 2.4).

CASE 2.4 Pharmacoresistance?

A young woman has a right cerebri media infarction because of carotid dissection. She lives alone and is unfortunately not found until the next day, with a malignant media infarction under development. She undergoes hemicraniectomy, has acute symptomatic seizures and seizures after the first week, and undergoes extensive rehabilitation. Six months after the infarction she is discharged from rehab with a referral to neurology outpatient because of an unsatisfactory seizure situation.

The patient can walk with assistance and has no aphasia, but a left spastic hemiparesis. Her mother accompanies her to the visit and describes frequent—often weekly—focal motor seizures which causes the patient to fall to the ground. There is impaired consciousness and the patient often takes 15 minutes to recover. She was started on phenytoin while in neurosurgical care, which was switched to carbamazepine in rehabilitation. She is now on 400 mg bid and reports no side effects.

Levetiracetam is added and increased to 1500 mg bid, with the immediate effect that seizures become less frequent and less severe—there is most often preserved consciousness and no falls. Carbamazepine (slow release) is next switched to oxcarbazepine. The patient became largely seizure free; occasional seizures are reported at missed doses.

> *Comment: The case illustrates several aspects of poststroke epilepsy. Medically, the patient has a severe stroke and a very short latency to seizure onset, indicating that she has several risk factors for pharmacoresistance. Despite this fact, revision of the initial therapy improves the situation considerably. Oxcarbazepine has less enzyme-inducing effect than carbamazepine (although not negligible), which may be beneficial. Finally, the case illustrates that the patient's seizure situation was probably not managed ambitiously enough throughout rehabilitation, which is also not uncommon.*

2.6.2 Quality of Life

Poststroke epilepsy can have an impact on quality of life. Methodologically, this effect is difficult to separate from the effects of stroke itself, especially since patients with more severe strokes are the ones who tend to develop epilepsy. In one of the larger studies demonstrating low quality of life associated with poststroke epilepsy, additional factors associated with reduced quality of life were seizure frequency and depression.[106] The German cohort was large and typical for poststroke epilepsy (mean age of 67, latency to the first seizure on average six months after the stroke). Initiation of ASM therapy resulted in relatively high proportions of side effects, including dizziness, nausea, and fatigue. Interestingly, these were reduced over the following two years, during which therapy was adapted and patients probably also familiarized with the therapy. At the end of the follow-up, 13% reported dizziness and 9% nausea, which were the more prominent side effects. Throughout the follow-up, patients with poststroke epilepsy had a worse trajectory regarding quality of life compared to patients without seizures after their stroke. Taken together, the literature underlines the importance of striving for seizure freedom and addressing psychiatric comorbidities in poststroke epilepsy, just like in any epilepsy.

2.6.3 Survival

Adequately powered studies suggest that poststroke epilepsy increases the risk of death.[10,107] Much of the literature suggesting otherwise is affected by survival bias, and many studies do not take into account immortalization effects (patients have to survive for some time to develop poststroke epilepsy). The reason for the excess mortality, which is of a magnitude of approximately 50% compared to stroke without subsequent epilepsy, is not known. Vascular causes seem more common than epilepsy-related ones.

TABLE 2.5   Clinical Take-Home Messages

- Epilepsy after stroke will develop in 6% after ischemic and 12% after hemorrhagic stroke.
- The risk of epilepsy is approximately 30% after an acute symptomatic seizure, but higher in cases of status epilepticus.
- The risk after late seizures can be above 60%.
- Seizures can mimic stroke or be acute symptomatic. Advanced imaging is often helpful in decisions about revascularization.
- Short latency to the first seizure increases the risk of pharmacoresistance.
- In treatment, it is important to avoid ASMs interacting with secondary stroke prophylaxis.
- Seizure freedom and depression influence quality of life in poststroke epilepsy.

In over 7000 patients with poststroke epilepsy in Sweden, vascular disease was the most common cause of death.[108] Contributors to detrimental vascular events may be that ASMs can interfere with stroke prophylaxis, that risk of seizures may hamper rehabilitation by deterring patients from physical activity, and that older antiepileptic drugs have negative effects on vascular health. Seizure-related risks could also play a role. Status epilepticus is not uncommon after stroke, afflicting 25% of cases in one series.[59] Nonetheless, seizures or SUDEP are probably not the direct cause in most deaths in persons with poststroke epilepsy. Pathophysiologically, the risk of SUDEP is mainly related to tonic-clonic seizures, and many seizures after stroke are focal.

The literature on survival with poststroke epilepsy suggests that vascular health is a very important factor that needs to be considered in epilepsy management (Table 2.5). Patients with poststroke epilepsy seem to be a vascular high-risk group. ASM treatment should therefore not interact with vascular drugs, and more focus on preventing vascular events will probably become more important in the neurological care of seizures after stroke in the future.

REFERENCES

1. Forsgren L, Beghi E, Oun A, Sillanpaa M. The epidemiology of epilepsy in Europe —a systematic review. Eur. J. Neurol. 2005 April;12:245–253.
2. Syvertsen M, Nakken KO, Edland A, Hansen G, Hellum MK, Koht J. Prevalence and etiology of epilepsy in a Norwegian county: a population based study. Epilepsia. 2015 May;56:699–706.
3. Lossius MI, Ronning OM, Mowinckel P, Gjerstad L. Incidence and predictors for post-stroke epilepsy: a prospective controlled trial. The Akershus stroke study. Eur. J. Neurol. 2002 July;9:365–368.
4. Kammersgaard LP, Olsen TS. Poststroke epilepsy in the Copenhagen stroke study: incidence and predictors. J. Stroke Cerebrovasc. Dis. 2005 September–October;14:210–214.
5. Bladin CF, Alexandrov AV, Bellavance A, Bornstein N, Chambers B, Cote R, et al. Seizures after stroke: a prospective multicenter study. Arch. Neurol. 2000 November;57:1617–1622.

6. Guo J, Guo J, Li J, Zhou M, Qin F, Zhang S, et al. Statin treatment reduces the risk of poststroke seizures. Neurology. 2015 August 25;85:701–707.

7. Burn J, Dennis M, Bamford J, Sandercock P, Wade D, Warlow C. Epileptic seizures after a first stroke: the Oxfordshire Community Stroke Project. BMJ. 1997 December 13;315:1582–1587.

8. Bryndziar T, Sedova P, Kramer NM, Mandrekar J, Mikulik R, Brown RD Jr, et al. Seizures following ischemic stroke: frequency of occurrence and impact on outcome in a long-term population-based study. J. Stroke Cerebrovasc. Dis. 2015 October 7;25:150–156.

9. Jungehulsing GJ, Heuschmann PU, Holtkamp M, Schwab S, Kolominsky-Rabas PL. Incidence and predictors of post-stroke epilepsy. Acta Neurol. Scand. 2013 June;127:427–430.

10. Zelano J, Redfors P, Asberg S, Kumlien E. Association between poststroke epilepsy and death: a nationwide cohort study. Eur. Stroke J. 2016 December;1:272–278. Original research article.

11. Lahti AM, Saloheimo P, Huhtakangas J, Salminen H, Juvela S, Bode MK, et al. Poststroke epilepsy in long-term survivors of primary intracerebral hemorrhage Neurology. 2017 June 6;88: 2169 –2175.

12. Graham NS, Crichton S, Koutroumanidis M, Wolfe CD, Rudd AG. Incidence and associations of poststroke epilepsy: the prospective South London Stroke Register. Stroke. 2013 March;44:605–611.

13. Pitkanen A, Roivainen R, Lukasiuk K. Development of epilepsy after ischaemic stroke Lancet Neurol. 2015 November 13;15:185–197.

14. Beghi E, Carpio A, Forsgren L, Hesdorffer DC, Malmgren K, Sander JW, et al. Recommendation for a definition of acute symptomatic seizure. Epilepsia. 2010 April;51:671–675.

15. Ferlazzo E, Gasparini S, Beghi E, Sueri C, Russo E, Leo A, et al. Epilepsy in cerebrovascular diseases: review of experimental and clinical data with meta-analysis of risk factors. Epilepsia. 2016 August;57:1205–1214.

16. Sinka L, Abraira L, Imbach LL, Zieglgansberger D, Santamarina E, Alvarez-Sabin J, et al. Association of mortality and risk of epilepsy with type of acute symptomatic seizure after ischemic stroke and an updated prognostic model. JAMA Neurol. 2023 June 1;80:605–613.

17. Lattanzi S, Meletti S, Trinka E, Brigo F, Turcato G, Rinaldi C, et al. Individualized prediction of drug resistance in people with post-stroke epilepsy: a retrospective study. J. Clin. Med. 2023 May 23;12:3610.

18. De Reuck J, Sieben A, Van Maele G. Characteristics and outcomes of patients with seizures according to the time of onset in relation to stroke. Eur. Neurol. 2008;59:225–228.

19. Lattanzi S, Orlandi N, Giovannini G, Brigo F, Trinka E, Meletti S. The risk of unprovoked seizure occurrence after status epilepticus in adults. Epilepsia. 2024 February 10;65:1006–1016.

20. Schaper F, Nordberg J, Cohen AL, Lin C, Hsu J, Horn A, et al. Mapping lesion-related epilepsy to a human brain network. JAMA Neurol. 2023 September 1;80:891–902.

21. Johnson EL, Krauss GL, Lee AK, Schneider ALC, Dearborn JL, Kucharska-Newton AM, et al. Association between midlife risk factors and late-onset epilepsy: results from the atherosclerosis risk in communities study. JAMA Neurol. 2018 November 1;75:1375–1382.

22. Doerrfuss JI, Hebel JM, Holtkamp M. Epileptogenicity of white matter lesions in cerebral small vessel disease: a systematic review and meta-analysis. J. Neurol. 2023 October;270:4890–4902.

23. Hlauschek G, Nicolo JP, Sinclair B, Law M, Yasuda CL, Cendes F, et al. Role of the glymphatic system and perivascular spaces as a potential biomarker for post-stroke epilepsy. Epilepsia Open. 2024 February;9:60–76.

24. Eriksson H, Wirdefeldt K, Asberg S, Zelano J. Family history increases the risk of late seizures after stroke. Neurology. 2019 November 19;93:e1964–e1970.

25. Zhang B, Chen M, Yang H, Wu T, Song C, Guo R. Evidence for involvement of the CD40/CD40L system in post-stroke epilepsy. Neurosci. Lett. 2014 May 1;567:6–10.

26. Yang H, Song Z, Yang GP, Zhang BK, Chen M, Wu T, et al. The ALDH2 rs671 polymorphism affects post-stroke epilepsy susceptibility and plasma 4-HNE levels. PLOS ONE. 2014;9:e109634.
27. Xie C, Sun J, Qiao W, Lu D, Wei L, Na M, et al. Administration of simvastatin after kainic acid-induced status epilepticus restrains chronic temporal lobe epilepsy. PLOS ONE. 2011;6:e24966.
28. van Vliet EA, Holtman L, Aronica E, Schmitz LJ, Wadman WJ, Gorter JA. Atorvastatin treatment during epileptogenesis in a rat model for temporal lobe epilepsy. Epilepsia. 2011 July;52:1319–1330.
29. Gouveia TL, Scorza FA, Iha HA, Frangiotti MI, Perosa SR, Cavalheiro EA, et al. Lovastatin decreases the synthesis of inflammatory mediators during epileptogenesis in the hippocampus of rats submitted to pilocarpine-induced epilepsy. Epilepsy Behav. 2014 July;36:68–73.
30. Pitkanen A, Kharatishvili I, Karhunen H, Lukasiuk K, Immonen R, Nairismagi J, et al. Epileptogenesis in experimental models. Epilepsia. 2007;48 Suppl 2:13–20.
31. Temkin NR. Antiepileptogenesis and seizure prevention trials with antiepileptic drugs: meta-analysis of controlled trials. Epilepsia. 2001 April;42:515–524.
32. Etminan M, Samii A, Brophy JM. Statin use and risk of epilepsy: a nested case-control study. Neurology. 2010 October 26;75:1496–1500.
33. Gensicke H, Seiffge DJ, Polasek AE, Peters N, Bonati LH, Lyrer PA, et al. Long-term outcome in stroke patients treated with IV thrombolysis. Neurology. 2013 March 5;80:919–925.
34. Tan ML, Ng A, Pandher PS, Sashindranath M, Hamilton JA, Davis SM, et al. Tissue plasminogen activator does not alter development of acquired epilepsy. Epilepsia. 2012 November;53:1998–2004.
35. Eriksson H, Nordanstig A, Rentzos A, Zelano J, Redfors P. Risk of poststroke epilepsy after reperfusion therapies: a national cohort study. Eur. J. Neurol. 2023 May;30:1303–1311.
36. Gilad R, Boaz M, Dabby R, Sadeh M, Lampl Y. Are post intracerebral hemorrhage seizures prevented by anti-epileptic treatment ? Epilepsy Res. 2011 August;95: 227 –231.
37. Peter-Derex L, Philippeau F, Garnier P, Andre-Obadia N, Boulogne S, Catenoix H, et al. Safety and efficacy of prophylactic levetiracetam for prevention of epileptic seizures in the acute phase of intracerebral haemorrhage (PEACH): a randomised, double-blind, placebo-controlled, phase 3 trial. Lancet Neurol. 2022 September;21:781–791.
38. Zhu Y, Gou H, Ma L, Sun J, Hou Y, Li Y, et al. Effects of double-dose statin therapy for the prevention of post-stroke epilepsy: a prospective clinical study. Seizure. 2021 May;88:138–142.
39. Passero S, Rocchi R, Rossi S, Ulivelli M, Vatti G. Seizures after spontaneous supratentorial intracerebral hemorrhage. Epilepsia. 2002 October;43:1175–1180.
40. Ebbesen MQB, Dreier JW, Lolk K, Andersen G, Johnsen SP, Zelano J, et al. Revascularization therapies for ischemic stroke and association with risk of epilepsy: a Danish Nationwide Register-Based Study. J. Am. Heart Assoc. 2024 August 6;13:e034279.
41. Abraira L, Santamarina E, Cazorla S, Bustamante A, Quintana M, Toledo M, et al. Blood biomarkers predictive of epilepsy after an acute stroke event. Epilepsia. 2020 October;61:2244–2253.
42. Abraira L, Giannini N, Santamarina E, Cazorla S, Bustamante A, Quintana M, et al. Correlation of blood biomarkers with early-onset seizures after an acute stroke event Epilepsy Behav. 2020 March;104:106549.
43. Eriksson H, Lowhagen Henden P, Rentzos A, Pujol-Calderon F, Karlsson JE, Hoglund K, et al. Acute symptomatic seizures and epilepsy after mechanical thrombectomy. Epilepsy Behav. 2019 September 13;104:106520.
44. Eriksson H, Banote RK, Larsson D, Blennow K, Zetterberg H, Zelano J. Brain injury markers in new-onset seizures in adults: a pilot study. Seizure. 2021 November;92:62–67.

45. Galovic M, Ferreira-Atuesta C, Abraira L, Dohler N, Sinka L, Brigo F, et al. Seizures and epilepsy after stroke: epidemiology. Biomark. Manag. Drugs Aging. 2021 April;38:285–299.
46. Bentes C, Martins H, Peralta AR, Casimiro C, Morgado C, Franco AC, et al. Post-stroke seizures are clinically underestimated. J. Neurol. 2017 September;264:1978–1985.
47. Shinton RA, Gill JS, Zezulka AV, Beevers DG. The frequency of epilepsy preceding stroke: case-control study in 230 patients. Lancet. 1987 January 3;1:11–13.
48. Zelano J, Larsson D, Kumlien E, Asberg S. Pre-stroke seizures: a nationwide register-based investigation. Seizure. 2017 July;49:25–29.
49. Larsson D, Farahmand B, Asberg S, Zelano J. Risk of stroke after new-onset seizures. Seizure. 2020 October 5;83:76–82.
50. Galovic M, Dohler N, Erdelyi-Canavese B, Felbecker A, Siebel P, Conrad J, et al. Prediction of late seizures after ischaemic stroke with a novel prognostic model (the SeLECT score): a multivariable prediction model development and validation study. Lancet Neurol. 2018 February;17:143–152.
51. Haapaniemi E, Strbian D, Rossi C, Putaala J, Sipi T, Mustanoja S, et al. The CAVE score for predicting late seizures after intracerebral hemorrhage. Stroke J. Cereb. Circ. 2014 July;45:1971–1976.
52. Arboix A, Garcia-Eroles L, Massons JB, Oliveres M, Comes E. Predictive factors of early seizures after acute cerebrovascular disease. Stroke J. Cereb. Circ. 1997 August;28:1590–1594.
53. De Herdt V, Dumont F, Henon H, Derambure P, Vonck K, Leys D, et al. Early seizures in intracerebral hemorrhage: incidence, associated factors, and outcome. Neurology. 2011 November 15;77:1794–1800.
54. Labovitz DL, Hauser WA, Sacco RL. Prevalence and predictors of early seizure and status epilepticus after first stroke. Neurology. 2001 July 24;57:200–206.
55. Kilpatrick CJ, Davis SM, Hopper JL, Rossiter SC. Early seizures after acute stroke: risk of late seizures. Arch. Neurol. 1992 May;49:509–511.
56. Hesdorffer DC, Benn EK, Cascino GD, Hauser WA. Is a first acute symptomatic seizure epilepsy? Mortality and risk for recurrent seizure. Epilepsia. 2009 May;50:1102–1108.
57. Fisher RS, Acevedo C, Arzimanoglou A, Bogacz A, Cross JH, Elger CE, et al. ILAE official report: a practical clinical definition of epilepsy. Epilepsia. 2014 April;55:475–482.
58. Zelano J. Recurrence risk after a first remote symptomatic seizure in adults: epilepsy or not? Epilepsia Open. 2021 December;6:634–644.
59. Zelano J, Lundberg RG, Baars L, Hedegard E, Kumlien E. Clinical course of poststroke epilepsy: a retrospective nested case-control study. Brain Behav. 2015 September;5:e00366.
60. Huttunen J, Kurki MI, von Und Zu Fraunberg M, Koivisto T, Ronkainen A, Rinne J, et al. Epilepsy after aneurysmal subarachnoid hemorrhage: a population-based, long-term follow-up study. Neurology. 2015 June 2;84:2229–2237.
61. Kotila M, Waltimo O. Epilepsy after stroke. Epilepsia. 1992 May–June;33:495–498.
62. Gilmore E, Choi HA, Hirsch LJ, Claassen J. Seizures and CNS hemorrhage: spontaneous intracerebral and aneurysmal subarachnoid hemorrhage. Neurologist. 2010 May;16:165–175.
63. Lindgren E, Silvis SM, Hiltunen S, Heldner MR, Serrano F, de Scisco M, et al. Acute symptomatic seizures in cerebral venous thrombosis. Neurology. 2020 September 22;95:e1706–e1715.
64. Sanchez van Kammen M, Lindgren E, Silvis SM, Hiltunen S, Heldner MR, Serrano F, et al. Late seizures in cerebral venous thrombosis. Neurology. 2020 September 22;95:e1716–e1723.
65. Bauer G, Trinka E. Nonconvulsive status epilepticus and coma. Epilepsia. 2010 February;51:177–190.
66. Westhall E, Rundgren M, Lilja G, Friberg H, Cronberg T. Postanoxic status epilepticus can be identified and treatment guided successfully by continuous electroencephalography. Ther. Hypotherm. Temp. Manag. 2013 June;3:84–87.

67. Rossetti AO, Oddo M, Liaudet L, Kaplan PW. Predictors of awakening from postanoxic status epilepticus after therapeutic hypothermia. Neurology. 2009 February 24;72:744–749.

68. Sutter R, Marsch S, Fuhr P, Ruegg S. Mortality and recovery from refractory status epilepticus in the intensive care unit: a 7-year observational study. Epilepsia. 2013 March;54:502–511.

69. Ruijter BJ, Keijzer HM, Tjepkema-Cloostermans MC, Blans MJ, Beishuizen A, Tromp SC, et al. Treating rhythmic and periodic EEG patterns in comatose survivors of cardiac arrest. N. Engl. J. Med. 2022 February 24;386:724–734.

70. Nolan JP, Sandroni C, Bottiger BW, Cariou A, Cronberg T, Friberg H, et al. European Resuscitation Council and European Society of Intensive Care Medicine Guidelines 2021: post-resuscitation care. Resuscitation. 2021 April;161:220–269.

71. Lance JW, Adams RD. The syndrome of intention or action myoclonus as a sequel to hypoxic encephalopathy. Brain J. Neurol. 1963 March;86:111–136.

72. Brochner AC, Lindholm P, Jensen MJ, Toft P, Henriksen FL, Lassen JF, et al. Post-hypoxic myoclonus status following out-of-hospital cardiac arrest-does it still predict a poor outcome? A retrospective study. Healthcare (Basel). 2021 December 27;10.

73. Elmer J, Rittenberger JC, Faro J, Molyneaux BJ, Popescu A, Callaway CW, et al. Clinically distinct electroencephalographic phenotypes of early myoclonus after cardiac arrest. Ann. Neurol. 2016 August;80:175–184.

74. Morris NA, May TL, Motta M, Agarwal S, Kamel H. Long-term risk of seizures among cardiac arrest survivors. Resuscitation. 2018 August;129:94–96.

75. Shaker H, Milan A, Alsallom F, Newey C, Hantus S, Punia V. Long-term electro-clinical profile of sudden cardiac arrest survivors. Epilepsia Open. 2021 September;6:559–568.

76. Polymeris AA, Curtze S, Erdur H, Hametner C, Heldner MR, Groot AE, et al. Intravenous thrombolysis for suspected ischemic stroke with seizure at onset. Ann. Neurol. 2019 November;86:770–779.

77. De Reuck J, De Groote L, Van Maele G. Single seizure and epilepsy in patients with a cerebral territorial infarct. J. Neurol. Sci. 2008 August 15;271:127–130.

78. Fukuma K, Ikeda S, Tanaka T, Kamogawa N, Ishiyama H, Abe S, et al. Clinical and imaging features of nonmotor onset seizure in poststroke epilepsy. Epilepsia. 2022 August;63:2068–2080.

79. Sylaja PN, Dzialowski I, Krol A, Roy J, Federico P, Demchuk AM, et al. Role of CT angiography in thrombolysis decision-making for patients with presumed seizure at stroke onset. Stroke J. Cereb. Circ. 2006 March;37:915–917.

80. Bogousslavsky J, Martin R, Regli F, Despland PA, Bolyn S. Persistent worsening of stroke sequelae after delayed seizures. Arch. Neurol. 1992 April;49:385–388.

81. De Reuck J, Claeys I, Martens S, Vanwalleghem P, Van Maele G, Phlypo R, et al. Computed tomographic changes of the brain and clinical outcome of patients with seizures and epilepsy after an ischaemic hemispheric stroke. Eur. J. Neurol. 2006 April;13:402–407.

82. De Reuck J, Vanhee F, Van Maele G, Claeys I. Magnetic resonance imaging after seizures in patients with an ischemic stroke. Cerebrovasc. Dis. 2007;23:339–343.

83. Zaccara G, Lattanzi S, Brigo F. Acute symptomatic seizures after stroke: a scoping review on primary prevention, treatment with antiseizure medications and drug discontinuation. Epilepsy Behav. 2023 December;149:109499.

84. Zelano J, Holtkamp M, Agarwal N, Lattanzi S, Trinka E, Brigo F. How to diagnose and treat post-stroke seizures and epilepsy. Epileptic Disord. 2020 June 1;22:252–263.

85. Hesdorffer DC, Logroscino G, Cascino G, Annegers JF, Hauser WA. Risk of unprovoked seizure after acute symptomatic seizure: effect of status epilepticus. Ann. Neurol. 1998 December;44:908–912.

86. Velioglu SK, Ozmenoglu M, Boz C, Alioglu Z. Status epilepticus after stroke. Stroke J. Cereb. Circ. 2001 May;32:1169–1172.

87. Lekoubou A, Wu EY, Bishu KG, Ovbiagele B. Prevalence, predictors, and prognosis of mortality among elderly stroke patients with convulsive status epilepticus in the United States. J. Neurol. Sci. 2022 September 15;440:120342.
88. Mintzer S, Trinka E, Kraemer G, Chervoneva I, Werhahn KJ. Impact of carbamazepine, lamotrigine, and levetiracetam on vascular risk markers and lipid-lowering agents in the elderly. Epilepsia. 2018 October;59:1899–1907.
89. Falcao A, Pinto R, Nunes T, Soares-da-Silva P. Effect of repeated administration of eslicarbazepine acetate on the pharmacokinetics of simvastatin in healthy subjects Epilepsy Res. 2013 September;106: 244 –249.
90. Vyas MV, Davidson BA, Escalaya L, Costella J, Saposnik G, Burneo JG. Antiepileptic drug use for treatment of epilepsy and dyslipidemia: systematic review. Epilepsy Res. 2015 July;113:44–67.
91. Larsson D, Baftiu A, Johannessen Landmark C, von Euler M, Kumlien E, Asberg S, et al. Association between antiseizure drug monotherapy and mortality for patients with poststroke epilepsy. JAMA Neurol. 2022 February 1;79:169–175.
92. Katsiki N, Mikhailidis DP, Nair DR. The effects of antiepileptic drugs on vascular risk factors: a narrative review. Seizure. 2014 October;23:677–684.
93. Werhahn KJ, Trinka E, Dobesberger J, Unterberger I, Baum P, Deckert-Schmitz M, et al. A randomized, double-blind comparison of antiepileptic drug treatment in the elderly with new-onset focal epilepsy. Epilepsia. 2015 March;56:450–459.
94. Werhahn KJ, Klimpe S, Balkaya S, Trinka E, Kramer G. The safety and efficacy of add-on levetiracetam in elderly patients with focal epilepsy: a one-year observational study. Seizure. 2011 May;20:305–311.
95. Pohlmann-Eden B, Marson AG, Noack-Rink M, Ramirez F, Tofighy A, Werhahn KJ, et al. Comparative effectiveness of levetiracetam, valproate and carbamazepine among elderly patients with newly diagnosed epilepsy: subgroup analysis of the randomized, unblinded KOMET study. BMC Neurol. 2016 August 23;16:149.
96. Marson AG, Al-Kharusi AM, Alwaidh M, Appleton R, Baker GA, Chadwick DW, et al. The SANAD study of effectiveness of carbamazepine, gabapentin, lamotrigine, oxcarbazepine, or topiramate for treatment of partial epilepsy: an unblinded randomised controlled trial. Lancet. 2007 March 24;369:1000–1015.
97. Kutlu G, Gomceli YB, Unal Y, Inan LE. Levetiracetam monotherapy for late poststroke seizures in the elderly. Epilepsy Behav. 2008 October;13:542–544.
98. Gilad R, Sadeh M, Rapoport A, Dabby R, Boaz M, Lampl Y. Monotherapy of lamotrigine versus carbamazepine in patients with poststroke seizure. Clin. Neuropharmacol. 2007 July–August;30:189–195.
99. Consoli D, Bosco D, Postorino P, Galati F, Plastino M, Perticoni GF, et al. Levetiracetam versus carbamazepine in patients with late poststroke seizures: a multicenter prospective randomized open-label study (EpIC project). Cerebrovasc. Dis. 2012;34:282–289.
100. Brigo F, Lattanzi S, Zelano J, Bragazzi NL, Belcastro V, Nardone R, et al. Randomized controlled trials of antiepileptic drugs for the treatment of post-stroke seizures: a systematic review with network meta-analysis. Seizure. 2018 October;61:57–62.
101. Alvarez-Sabin J, Montaner J, Padro L, Molina CA, Rovira R, Codina A, et al. Gabapentin in late-onset poststroke seizures. Neurology. 2002 December 24;59:1991–1993.
102. Larsson D, Asberg S, Kumlien E, Zelano J. Retention rate of first antiepileptic drug in poststroke epilepsy: a nationwide study. Seizure. 2019 January;64:29–33.
103. Beghi E, Giussani G, Grosso S, Iudice A, La Neve A, Pisani F, et al. Withdrawal of antiepileptic drugs: guidelines of the Italian League Against Epilepsy. Epilepsia. 2013 October;54 Suppl 7:2–12.
104. Silverman IE, Restrepo L, Mathews GC. Poststroke seizures. Arch. Neurol. 2002 February; 59:195–201.

105. Redfors P, Holmegaard L, Pedersen A, Jern C, Malmgren K. Long-term follow-up of post-stroke epilepsy after ischemic stroke: room for improved epilepsy treatment. Seizure. 2020 January 21;76:50–55.

106. Winter Y, Daneshkhah N, Galland N, Kotulla I, Kruger A, Groppa S. Health-related quality of life in patients with poststroke epilepsy. Epilepsy Behav. 2018 March;80:303–306.

107. Arntz RM, Rutten-Jacobs LC, Maaijwee NA, Schoonderwaldt HC, Dorresteijn LD, van Dijk EJ, et al. Poststroke epilepsy is associated with a high mortality after a stroke at young age: follow-up of transient ischemic attack and stroke patients and unelucidated risk factor evaluation study. Stroke J. Cereb. Circ. 2015 August;46:2309–2311.

108. Hansen J, Asberg S, Kumlien E, Zelano J. Cause of death in patients with poststroke epilepsy: results from a nationwide cohort study. PLOS ONE. 2017;12:e0174659.

Post-traumatic Epilepsy

3

3.1 RISK OF EPILEPSY

Traumatic brain injury accounts for approximately 5% of epilepsy worldwide and remains one of the common causes of epilepsy, particularly in developing countries.[1] With ageing populations, cerebrovascular disease has probably surpassed traumatic brain injury as an epilepsy etiology in most countries, but because traumatic brain injury often affects young persons, post-traumatic epilepsy is prevalent and frequently encountered in clinical practice. It is also a significant contributor to the global burden of epilepsy in terms of morbidity.

3.1.1 Prevalence

The prevalence of post-traumatic epilepsy in a country or region is influenced by the risk of traumatic brain injury and the type of injury. For instance, the United States has a higher number of traumatic brain injuries per year than Europe.[2] The risk is particularly high after penetrating head injuries, which means that countries with many gunshot victims or war veterans may have higher prevalence. Some of the studies showing the highest risk of post-traumatic epilepsy are on veterans from the Vietnam or Iran–Iraq wars, where detailed follow-up is available for large cohorts with severe brain injury.[3,4] The prevalence in civilian populations is naturally much lower. In a Norwegian population-based study on epilepsy etiology, trauma accounted for 13% of all structural epilepsy and 6% of all epilepsy in the population.[5]

3.1.2 Incidence

Reported absolute risks of post-traumatic epilepsy range from 2% to 50% depending on the study setting. The severity of the trauma is the major risk factor—Annegers found that 2.1% developed epilepsy after mild, 4.2% after moderate, and 16.7% after severe traumatic brain injury.[6] In Swedish adults hospitalized for traumatic brain injury in

DOI: 10.1201/9781003501404-3

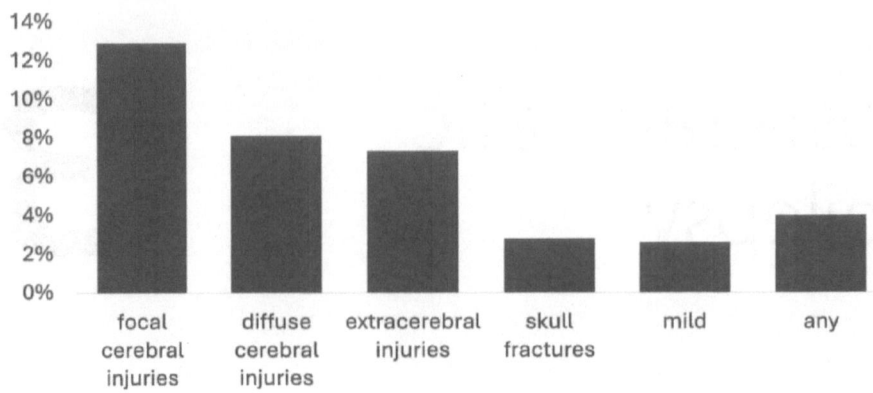

FIGURE 3.1   Cumulative 10-year incidence of post-traumatic epilepsy after different injury types.[7]

2000–2010 the 10-year risks were 13% for focal cerebral injuries, 7%–8% for diffuse or extracerebral injuries, and 2.8% for mild traumatic brain injury (Figure 3.1).[7]

The risk of developing epilepsy decreases with time after a traumatic brain injury, like for most acquired epilepsies.[7,8] The risk is highest in year one after the trauma, but after five years the annual risk of developing epilepsy drops below 1%.[2] However, many studies report that the risk of epilepsy continues to be slightly elevated compared to controls for years after the brain injury.[1,9] Whether this represents repeated trauma, unknown factors that also increase the risk of epilepsy, or neurobiological processes started by the initial trauma is not known. There are complicated confounders in the study of long-term risks of post-traumatic epilepsy; for instance, there may be risk factors common to epilepsy and traumatic brain injury.

CASE 3.1 Long Latency

A 32-year-old male is referred after two episodes of loss of consciousness. He remembers nothing of these except waking up with his girlfriend beside him. She describes how he turned to the right, became stiff, fell to the ground, and shook violently for a minute or so on the first occasion. On the second, she just heard him fall in a locked bathroom, after that there were thrashing sounds and once she was able to open the door he was unconscious but breathing heavily just like after the first occasion. In addition to these events, the patient reports that three years ago, he fell and sustained a head injury while out hiking. He was admitted to a hospital where he was told he had had a seizure. He doesn't remember anything from this episode except having muscle ache the day after being admitted to the hospital and headache. Review of the records shows that admission CT showed bilateral frontobasal bleeding (contusion). He is diagnosed with epilepsy and started on levetiracetam. A new MRI shows gliosis in the area of the contusions on the CT three years ago.

> *Comment: The case illustrates the uncertainty regarding epileptogenesis in post-traumatic epilepsy. In the episode three years ago, it is perhaps most likely that the patient suffered head trauma first and then an acute symptomatic seizure. Alternatively, he had a first seizure and sustained the injury, but three years of seizure freedom after that does not seem typical. On the other hand, three years is a long latency for post-traumatic epilepsy after a first acute symptomatic seizure. It is clear (see Epileptogenesis section) that a better understanding of trauma and risk of epilepsy is needed.*

3.2 EPILEPTOGENESIS

There are many clues to the mechanisms of epileptogenesis of post-traumatic epilepsy from animal and clinical studies, but actual biomarkers that can be used clinically have not been identified. Penetrating injuries affecting the cortex are more likely to cause epilepsy than diffuse or extracerebral injuries. There are conflicting results about whether the anatomic localization influences the risk, but at least some studies report that temporal lobe injury is associated with a greater risk.[10]

In animals, post-traumatic epilepsy is one of the more frequently studied epilepsies because of the robustness of animal models.[11] Impact injuries of various kinds are replicable and reliable producers of epilepsy. Following moderate and severe injury, there is axonal damage, inflammation, sprouting, and remodeling of neuronal networks. Plausible epileptogenesis mechanisms involved are also plasticity on a synapse level, inflammation, and perhaps genetic vulnerability.[12] In most models, inflammation seems to be a major driver of epileptogenesis, and antibodies blocking immune cells, other anti-inflammatory treatments, and ASMs can modulate epileptogenesis.

Despite apparently robust models, there has been no successful translation to clinic regarding biomarkers. With the rise of affordable proteomics, large international consortia have been formed that gather human clinical data for biomarker identification in parallel with animal modeling.[13] It remains to be seen whether the strategy will be successful. A problem with traumatic brain injury in humans is the large clinical variability, including not only the initial trauma but also secondary injuries and various neurosurgical interventions.

Epileptogenesis seems to have a highly variable time span in humans. Many patients develop post-traumatic epilepsy in the first year after traumatic brain injury, but the risk is increased beyond that albeit to a lesser degree. Conversely, there is evidence that epilepsy susceptibility can arise early; early seizures are a risk factor for subsequent epilepsy. In keeping with the notion of early epileptogenesis, it seems that admission EEG can be used for risk stratification; quantitative EEG analysis found that patients who later developed epilepsy had higher spectral power in the delta frequencies and more variance in other frequencies, again arguing for early indicators of at least vulnerability for epilepsy.[14]

Danish researchers have observed that a family history increases the epilepsy risk slightly, which raises the issue of genetic vulnerability.[15] The influence is likely to be minor compared to the injury characteristics but could exist to some degree. A systematic review found only four publications describing genetic markers increasing the risk of post-traumatic epilepsy, located in four genes.[16] The first encodes interleukin 1beta, a pro-inflammatory cytokine secreted by microglia and astrocytes. The other genes were glutamic acid decarboxylase 1 (GAD1), adenosine A1 receptor, which is highly expressed in hippocampus and cortex, and methylenetetrahydrofolate reductase (MTHFR), an enzyme used in processing of methionine. More research is needed, but it is interesting that both epidemiological and genetic research suggest the possibility of genetic vulnerability influencing the risk of post-traumatic epilepsy.

Another interesting aspect is the effect of repeated head trauma and age. Repeated head trauma increases the risk[17] and although the risk of epilepsy is highest after severe trauma, mild trauma also seems to increase the risk compared to the general population.[1] Regarding age, it is unclear if the findings reflect survival or if plasticity and network reorganization is more active in younger individuals.

3.2.1 Biomarkers and Antiepileptogenesis

Epileptogenesis after traumatic brain injury could perhaps be amendable to modulation of the risk. For instance, the risk of post-traumatic epilepsy seems increased in individuals using SSRI at the time of the traumatic brain injury.[18] This could reflect modulatory effect of the drugs or confounding by the underlying psychiatric indication.

Biomarkers of epileptogenesis after traumatic brain injury would be clinically very useful. Such markers would allow better surveillance for seizures, early treatment, and in the longer run perhaps antiepileptogenic therapeutic interventions. There have been attempts to better understand epileptogenesis by imaging and EEG. Imaging studies have included searching for blood–brain barrier disruption with CT or MRI, identification of inflammation by PET, gliosis and excitotoxic processes by MRI spectroscopy, and rearrangement of neural networks by fMRI.[19] Results have so far varied. An interesting novel avenue of research is perivascular spaces, which seem to be different in patients with post-traumatic epilepsy compared to traumatic brain injury only.[20] Whether the finding reflects post-traumatic changes leading to epilepsy or are a result of seizures is unknown.

EEG is another potential biomarker that seems to hold interesting potential. A systematic review has recently described how the field has evolved from single short EEG recordings to continuous EEG monitoring.[21] At the moment, there have been both studies finding that epileptiform discharges and/or slowing are not associated with later development of post-traumatic epilepsy and studies showing the opposite. If continuous EEG is used in intensive care, up to 35% of patients with traumatic brain injury will exhibit epileptiform activity or other pathological patterns.[22] Data on the prognostic significance of these patterns are not yet available.

There have been trials attempting to stop epileptogenesis with ASMs (Table 3.1). So far, they have been negative. In animals, modest advances have been made, but in

TABLE 3.1 Antiepileptogenesis, Selected Studies Trying to Prevent Post-traumatic Epilepsy

SELECTED STUDIES ON ANTIEPILEPTOGENESIS	
RANDOMIZED TRIALS	
STUDY	RESULT
Young et al. 1983[23]	Phenytoin did not reduce the rate of epilepsy compared to placebo.
Temkin et al. 1990[24]	Phenytoin reduced early, but not late, post-traumatic seizures more than placebo.
OBSERVATIONAL STUDIES	
STUDY	RESULT
Wilson 2018[25]	Meta-analysis. Levetiracetam and phenytoin decrease the risk of early seizures, but not subsequent epilepsy.

humans three trials have been negative so far, all using phenytoin.[23,26,27] Similarly, observational trials studying the effect of ASMs like levetiracetam or phenytoin during acute neurosurgical care on the later risk of post-traumatic epilepsy have not found any reduction in later epilepsy risk.[25,28] Future studies will probably try to study more enriched populations to reduce variability and thereby the needed sample size. Feasibility of a levetiracetam study aiming to prevent post-traumatic epilepsy has been demonstrated in children.[29]

3.3 RISK FACTORS

The severity of the injury is the most important risk factor of post-traumatic epilepsy (Table 3.2). In a Danish study of young adults and children, the relative risk of brain injury was increased 2.2 times after mild head injury compared to 7.4 times after severe brain injury.[15] Similar associations with injury severity have also been reported from the US and Sweden.[6,7,30] Different studies use different markers of injury severity, but regardless of whether these are the need for intensive care, level of consciousness, or imaging, the association with greater risks of post-traumatic epilepsy persists. Penetrating injuries constitute a particular risk. In a long-term study of Vietnam combat veterans with penetrating head injuries, half of the cohort developed post-traumatic epilepsy.[31]

Other risk factors include age, sex, other lesion characteristics, perhaps family history, and comorbidities. The findings vary, which is not surprising given that epilepsy and traumatic brain injury are common entities, making statistical analyses more challenging. Frequently identified risk factors include early seizures, subdural hematoma, skull fracture, loss of consciousness, and an age of 65 years or older.[6,30] In a Danish study of young adults and children, the risk increased more in persons older than 15 years at the time of the trauma and women had higher risk than men, as did persons with

TABLE 3.2   Some Risk Factors of Post-traumatic Epilepsy

Injury severity
Age
Hematoma and lesion characteristics
Comorbidities
Early seizures

a family history of epilepsy.[15] The finding regarding age should not be interpreted as children not having an increased risk of epilepsy after traumatic brain injury, but could reflect different injury severity—after mild traumatic brain injury one study found a cumulative incidence of post-traumatic epilepsy of 3.7%.[32] Conflicting results exist also for sex. In contrast to the Danish results cited earlier, a systematic review found that men had 1.3 times the risk of women.[8] Other risk factors were alcohol abuse, loss of consciousness, skull fracture, and different forms of structural brain injury visible on imaging. Age, early seizures, and severity of trauma were again identified as risk factors in a recent study of US insurance data.[33]

A recent investigation found hospital-acquired infections to be a risk factor for post-traumatic epilepsy.[34] This is an interesting notion, perhaps hinting at immune mechanisms adding to a pro-epileptogenic environment. There is naturally the risk of confounding of the severity of the trauma and more research is needed. If confirmed, it may indicate that particular vigilance needs to be applied in preventing hospital-acquired infections to reduce the risk of later epilepsy in traumatic brain injury patients.

3.4 RISKS AFTER THE FIRST SEIZURE

The literature on seizure recurrence is more heterogeneous in the field of traumatic brain injury than in poststroke epilepsy, perhaps because the most severe traumatic brain injuries are encountered in neurosurgery rather than neurology. Nonetheless, the same overall pattern emerges. It is important to distinguish acute symptomatic seizures (which may not necessarily indicate epilepsy) from later unprovoked seizures (which have a high recurrence risk).

3.4.1 Risk after an Acute Symptomatic Seizure

Early seizures occur within the first week of the trauma. This happens in approximately 2% of traumatic brain injury in population-based studies and in 14%–30% in selected cohorts with more severe traumatic brain injury.[2] After a first acute symptomatic seizure, the risk of a later unprovoked seizure is approximately 18%, meaning that most persons with a first acute symptomatic seizure will not develop unprovoked seizures.[35] It needs to be emphasized and explained to patients that although acute symptomatic seizures do not indicate epilepsy, they are a risk factor for subsequent epilepsy; the risk is higher than for persons that did not have a seizure during the first week after traumatic brain injury.[35]

3.4.2 Risks after a First Unprovoked Seizure

With the new ILAE clinical definition of epilepsy, allowing a diagnosis already after one seizure if the recurrence risk is high, many have attempted to identify traumatic brain injury cases in which a first unprovoked seizure indicates epilepsy. Until recently, the results have not been entirely clear (Figure 3.2). In a classic study on first seizures in 1955–1984 after traumatic brain injury involving loss of consciousness or amnesia for 30 minutes, skull fracture, or intracranial bleeding, the risk of a second unprovoked seizure was 47% (95% CI 30%–66%).[35] The small study population ($n = 37$) consisted of both children and adults, but regardless of these drawbacks, the result indicates that all unprovoked seizures after moderate TBI do not indicate epilepsy. A Swedish register-based investigation—interesting because of the predominantly non-gun-related injury panorama—found that the risk of epilepsy after a first seizure was clearly linked to trauma severity but could not identify any particular trauma group in which a first seizure indicated epilepsy to the certainty required by the ILAE.[36] Finally, studies on very severe injury populations, like patients admitted to US neurosurgical level 1 trauma centers (see Management section later for details) have reported that the risk of a second seizure after a first unprovoked seizure was at least 80%.[37] It therefore seems likely that in the most severe traumatic brain injury cases, a first late seizure could signify epilepsy. Indeed, a large US study recently showed that a single late seizure after severe traumatic brain injury has a recurrence risk of 82%.[38]

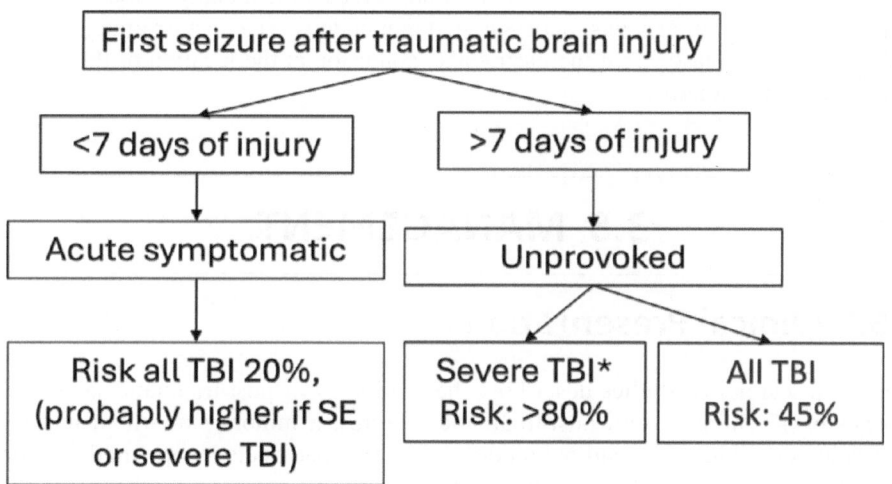

FIGURE 3.2   Risk of epilepsy after first seizures in different clinical situations.

Note: * Some studies indicate a very high risk after a first seizure in severe traumatic brain injury, perhaps motivating a diagnosis of epilepsy.

The latency between the trauma and the first late seizure does not seem to affect recurrence risk if the seizure occurs in the first two years.[37] First seizures occurring more than two years after the traumatic brain injury carries a lower risk of recurrence, at least according to Swedish patient register data using epilepsy diagnosis as a surrogate outcome.[36] That first seizures occurring later have a lower recurrence risk probably reflects that a proportion of these seizures are unrelated to the trauma and post-traumatic epileptogenic mechanisms. Ritter and co-workers have developed a predictive model, incorporating many of the most important risk factors.[39]

3.4.3 Risks after Other Injury Forms

3.4.3.1 Subdural Hematoma

A systematic review found that the cumulative incidence of post-traumatic epilepsy was 43% in acute SDH, and 10% in chronic SDH. Early seizures were present in 28% of acute SDH and 5% of chronic SDH. In acute SDH the most important risk factors of early or late seizures were low Glasgow Coma Scale (GCS) and craniotomy, whereas in chronic SDH alcohol abuse, altered mental status, previous stroke, and hematoma CT characteristics were most important.[40]

3.4.3.2 Craniotomy

Decompressive craniectomy is used in cases of trauma with raised intracranial pressure and is a frequently found risk factor of post-traumatic epilepsy. This may naturally be confounded by the severity of the initial trauma. A recent meta-analysis found the literature to be very heterogeneous, but suggested that epilepsy risk factors among patients undergoing cranioplasty were increasing age, contusion at the location of the surgery, and monopolar diathermy.[41]

3.5 MANAGEMENT

3.5.1 Clinical Presentation

There is a scarcity of studies describing the semiology of post-traumatic seizures. In a series of 47 children with post-traumatic seizures, a minority of whom had mild traumatic brain injury, the authors reported that 28% had acute symptomatic seizures within the first 24 hours of the trauma.[42] This mirrors the situation in other acute cerebral insults, like stroke, where acute symptomatic seizures usually occur early after the injury. Children with mild traumatic brain injury had both focal onset motor and focal onset non-motor seizures, as well as tonic-clonic seizures. In children with severe traumatic brain injury, there was a wider range of semiology (and more patients). Focal onset motor seizures and tonic-clonic seizures were most common, but some patients were reported to have epileptic spasms and hypomotor seizures.

In adults, a larger series of semiology has been reported for patients with intractable post-traumatic epilepsy after the Iran–Iraq war.[4] Ninety-seven patients had blunt head trauma and 66 had penetrating head trauma as their epilepsy etiology. Interestingly, the latency to the first seizure was shorter in patients with penetrating head trauma, underlining the very high epileptogenicity of this type of brain injury. There were no significant differences in seizure types between the two categories of brain injury. Focal onset seizures with and without loss of consciousness were most common, followed by bilateral tonic-clonic seizures. For patients with blunt head trauma, about one third had semiology that localized to the frontal lobe, and one third had semiology that localized to the temporal lobe. One third had seizures that were unlocalizable. In contrast, frontal and parietal lobe semiology were the most common seizure types in patients with penetrating head injury.

3.5.1.1 Sports-Related Convulsive Concussions

Convulsive concussion during sports is a distressing symptom that raises a number of questions immediately important for an athlete's career. The area is under-researched, and more knowledge is needed. A systematic review described a wide range of motor behaviors following the trauma, not all of which are necessarily epileptic seizures but may reflect disinhibition of brainstem/spinal cord structures in a manner similar to convulsive syncope. Bilateral/generalized tonic-clonic seizures movements were described in 34 (26%) of the identified 130 cases. Although the authors identified studies from a range of sports, boxing was particularly prevalent and nine boxers developed post-traumatic epilepsy.[43]

3.5.2 Estimating Recurrence Risk

When to start ASM treatment is an important question in post-traumatic cases, and estimating recurrence risk is key in counselling the patient. In cases of severe brain injury and seizures occurring more than one week after the trauma, the recurrence risk is certainly high. In the study cited earlier of 63 patients that had such late seizures after severe traumatic brain injury and were treated at a neurosurgery level 1 trauma center, further unprovoked seizures occurred in 86%.[37] The inclusion criteria indicated a severe traumatic brain injury: a depressed skull fracture, a penetrating head injury, a cortical contusion visible on CT, an acute intracranial hematoma, a GCS score of −<10, or an early seizure. A total of 71% of participants were comatose for more than seven days and 78% had cortical contusion visible on CT. The findings were later replicated in an observational study, showing that a first late seizure has a high recurrence risk after severe traumatic brain injury.[38] The severity of the traumatic brain injury in this study is further illustrated by the cumulative epilepsy incidence of 25% at five years. In summary, a first unprovoked seizure after very severe traumatic brain injury seems to suggest a high recurrence risk and can probably motivate epilepsy diagnosis as well as ASM treatment.

On the other hand, any seizure occurring more than seven days after any traumatic brain injury does not equal epilepsy. In the Rochester project, the recurrence risk was

46% for all traumatic brain injury, and in Swedish registers, the risk of epilepsy after a first admission for seizure was not at the recurrence risk of 60% mandated by the ILAE for an epilepsy diagnosis.[35,36] In intermediary cases it may sometimes be reasonable to offer ASM treatment, since the recurrence risk is high, but also to withhold the epilepsy diagnosis, since it is unclear if the recurrence risk is as high as demanded by the ILAE definition of epilepsy. Local traditions, guidelines, and patient preference are important factors in each management decision.

3.5.2.1 The Role of EEG

At the moment, the role of EEG in estimates of recurrence risk is complicated. Epileptiform activity on EEG in general means a higher recurrence risk. The problem is that in populations with other risk factors—like abnormal neurological examination and imaging abnormalities—the risk is already elevated above what is expected after a first unprovoked seizure.[44] How epileptiform activity relates to the other risk factors is unknown. In general, in cases of remote symptomatic etiology to first unprovoked seizures, the presence or absence of epileptiform activity on EEG does not add precision to the recurrence risk estimate, which is nonetheless high.[45] In cases of very severe traumatic brain injury, a first seizure indicates a high recurrence risk regardless of the EEG result, so in this case the investigation can probably be omitted.

3.5.3 Primary Prophylaxis

Some authorities in the neurosurgical field advocate primary prophylaxis for the prevention of early seizures in severe traumatic brain injury.[46] Neurosurgical practices vary, but randomized controlled trials have not found that phenytoin reduces the incidence of early seizures in severe head trauma in adults or children (Table 3.3).[47,48] The studies indicate that giving ASMs to broadly defined populations are unlikely to reduce the overall incidence of seizures. However, the studies do not really disprove the value of judicious neurosurgical use on a case-by-case basis—so the discussion is likely to continue. Despite an ongoing discussion, phenytoin has been used traditionally to prevent early seizures (seizures during the first week) following traumatic brain injury, and levetiracetam has become more popular recently. A global survey indicated that these two drugs are still the most commonly used but that practices vary widely.[49]

3.5.4 Treatment of Early Seizures

If treatment is considered motivated to reduce the risk of early seizures, it should be noted that such seizures often occur in the first 24 hours of the trauma, so prophylaxis is probably more effective if started immediately.[50] One study reported that patients with breakthrough seizures despite phenytoin prophylaxis were older and had more frequently undergone neurosurgery for hematoma evacuation.[51]

When selecting an ASM, levetiracetam has many advantages compared to older ASMs—not least a better side effect profile and fewer drug–drug interactions than

TABLE 3.3 Some Studies on Prevention of Early Seizures after Trauma

RANDOMIZED TRIALS	
STUDY	RESULT
Inaba et al. 2013[52]	No difference between levetiracetam and phenytoin in prevention of early seizures.
Young et al. 2004[48]	Phenytoin did not reduce the rate of early seizures in children compared to placebo.
Young et al. 1983[47]	Phenytoin did not reduce the rate of early seizures compared to placebo.
OBSERVATIONAL STUDIES	
STUDY	RESULT
Glaser et al. 2022[53]	No fewer early seizures (but better survival) in older adults who received ASMs in ICU.

phenytoin. Systematic reviews have not found any difference in the incidence of early seizures in patients given levetiracetam compared to patients given phenytoin, and one recent systematic review determined levetiracetam to be the more effective and safe choice.[27,52,54,55] This is in line with a study on craniotomy for non-traumatic causes, which may occasionally cause *de novo* seizures in a few percent of cases, that found levetiracetam better for prevention of seizures compared to phenytoin.[56] If a patient with traumatic brain injury develops an early seizure and treatment is considered necessary, the choice is often an ASM that can be administered quickly at a therapeutic dose. This explains the popularity of levetiracetam and phenytoin, but there are of course other ASMs with potential for intravenous loading.

As in other cases of early seizures, clinical judgment must be used to decide the duration of treatment. Patients need to be well informed of the risk of late unprovoked seizures, which is often low but not negligible. The risk of seizure recurrence after a first early post-traumatic seizure was only 13% (95% CI = 7%–25%) in adults and children in Rochester, Minnesota.[35] For severe traumatic brain injury the risk may be substantially higher, but clinical factors are not yet known that can more precisely identify patients with need for long-term ASM treatment. Should shared decision-making result in a decision of ASM withdrawal, slow tapering is best, since this may at least in theory mitigate the severity of seizures, should they arise.

3.5.5 Treatment of Epilepsy

There is not much information on any ASM being particularly well suited for post-traumatic epilepsy. This is surprising, given the substantial resources that have been put into research in the area in the past decades, but most efforts have been focused on risk factors and prevention. In fact, most pharmacological studies seem to have focused on preventing the first seizure after traumatic brain injury rather than treating epilepsy.[57] Most recommendations are not more specific than that any drug with the indication focal epilepsy may be used.[58] This reflects a lack of large comparative studies, so just like for any epilepsy, there is a need to tailor the medication to the characteristics of each patient.

What observational data exist suggest that newer-generation ASMs are superior to older ones, but data for brivaracetam, lacosamide, and other new drugs are currently missing. In a Swedish register-based analysis levetiracetam had a significantly higher retention than carbamazepine. The one-year retention rates were 80% (95% CI = 65%–89%) for levetiracetam, 77% (95% CI = 60%–88%) for lamotrigine, 65% (95% CI = 48%–78%) for valproic acid, and 62% (95% CI = 52%–70%) for carbamazepine, but only the difference between levetiracetam and carbamazepine was significant.[59] The study was entirely based on administrative data and provides only low-level evidence.

CASE 3.2 Side Effects

The patient in Case 3.1 with the frontal contusions becomes tired after starting levetiracetam and complains of irritability. He and his girlfriend interpret the symptoms mainly as related to stress from the diagnosis of epilepsy. For fear of losing driving ability, he sticks with the treatment for two years, despite being advised to switch. After a breakthrough seizure he agrees to switch to lamotrigine. The tiredness resolves, as do the mood problems.

> *Comment: Side effects can often be a more significant contributor to low quality of life than patients appreciate. Tiredness is a very individual side effect that should not be forgotten in young patients. Switching to another suitable ASM can be beneficial (levetiracetam and lamotrigine are mere examples; on a group level this is a realistic case but side effect sensitivity is always individual).*

3.5.6 Non-Medical Treatment

3.5.6.1 Epilepsy Surgery

Patients with post-traumatic epilepsy have sometimes been helped by epilepsy surgery, but success rates can be lower than in other etiologies.[60] Naturally, all epilepsy surgery is done on a case-by-case basis, so systematic evaluations are not available. In refractory cases, referral to surgical center may be warranted.

3.5.6.2 Psychosocial Support

Some literature suggests an overrepresentation of psychiatric comorbidities including post-traumatic stress, substance abuse, cognitive deficits, and psychosocial problems in persons with post-traumatic epilepsy. The generalizability of such observations is hard to determine, but in individual cases there may be a need for intervention targeting psychosocial factors. A systematic review of neuropsychological impairment found some congruence despite a very heterogeneous literature, suggesting that particular focus should be put on patients with pharmacoresistance and severe traumatic brain injury.[61]

Clinicians treating post-traumatic epilepsy need to be aware of the cognitive problems that can follow traumatic brain injury, like problems with memory, emotions, or executive function. Neuropsychological assessment if often helpful.

Some, but not all, studies find an association between post-traumatic seizures and short-term neuropsychological outcome, also when injury severity is taken into account.[62,63] Over a longer follow-up period post-traumatic epilepsy seems associated with a greater risk of cognitive problems or dementia than either head injury or epilepsy alone.[64] An interesting study comparing persons with post-traumatic epilepsy to persons with other epilepsy, stratified by drug resistance, found that patients with post-traumatic epilepsy have the most comorbidities and reported low quality of life. Drug-resistant epilepsy and post-traumatic epilepsy were associated with low quality of life, and particularly post-traumatic epilepsy was associated with a high burden of comorbidities.[65] The relationship between mental health issues and post-traumatic epilepsy is complex, perhaps because of shared risk factors or causal relationships. For instance, interesting studies have reported that mental health problems increase the risk of post-traumatic epilepsy, which in turn increases the risk of anxiety.[66] More research is needed on this bidirectional relationship. Importantly, post-traumatic epilepsy was identified as a predictor of anxiety and depression two years after traumatic brain injury.[66] The association was valid also with corrections for other predictors of poor mental health.

In summary, epilepsy and traumatic brain injury are both associated with a greater risk of neuropsychological problems.[49,62,66] For clinicians it is important to recognize the potential double vulnerability in patients with post-traumatic epilepsy and try to ensure adequate medical and social support. Such support may include extra contacts from the epilepsy nurse, social support workers, closer follow-up after diagnosis, and referral to psychiatric services. Neuropsychological evaluation is often important to make patients aware of deficits and allow compensatory strategies.

3.6 PROGNOSIS

Some case series of post-traumatic epilepsies suggest problems with pharmacoresistance, comorbidities, and psychosocial aspects. Whether this represents actual epilepsy refractoriness or cognitive or social problems after traumatic brain injury in turn affecting adherence is unknown. In children, one study found that 3/6 patients with post-traumatic epilepsy after mild traumatic brain injury became medically intractable.[32] Similar results have been reported from a population-based material in Korea, in which 14/34 patients with post-traumatic epilepsy (41%) were medically intractable.[67] Others have found pharmacoresistance in about one fifth of patients with post-traumatic epilepsy.[68,69] One of these studies used nearly 3000 patients to identify risk factors of drug resistance in post-traumatic epilepsy.[69] Out of several factors studied, four were associated with pharmacoresistance; age at post-traumatic epilepsy, seizure type, status epilepticus, and EEG findings (Table 3.4).

Some studies suggest an overrepresentation of substance abuse in patients with previous traumatic brain injury, highlighting that the population may in some cases have a complicated psychosocial situation.[7] In summary, it is well worth spending time in history taking on provoking factors and of course ASM adherence. When such reasons for treatment failure have been eliminated, it is important to treat post-traumatic epilepsy just as ambitiously as other epilepsy—therapy revision until remission or intolerable side effects.

In adults, mortality is about two-fold higher in patients with post-traumatic epilepsy than in patients that have not developed epilepsy after trauma.[70,71] Epilepsy and its treatment are likely to be part of the explanation. For all adults with post-traumatic epilepsy in Sweden, mortality was increased two-fold, but in the youngest age group the risk of death was nearly eight-fold higher than in age-matched controls.[72] Epilepsy was also a more common cause of death in younger age groups compared to older ones. The findings echo those in other investigations on post-traumatic epilepsy in which younger patients had higher death rates; adherence to ASM therapy and comorbidities were identified as important care elements.[73] In another Swedish population-based investigation, a traumatic epilepsy cause was associated with a more than a two-fold increased SUDEP risk compared to epilepsy of genetic cause.[74] This highlights the importance of monitoring SUDEP risk factors, particularly tonic-clonic seizures, and alerting patients to the potential consequences of poor adherence and guidance on prevention of seizure-related risks. Similarly, ensuring adequate support to help patients with medication adherence is fundamental.

It is possible that factors other than epilepsy account for some aspects of the increased mortality. An epidemiological study from Minnesota showed that the 10-year mortality did not differ between 30-day survivors of traumatic brain injury that had experienced an early seizure (21.7%, 95% CI 11.9%–37.5%) and 30-day survivors that had experienced a late post-traumatic seizure (28.1%, 95% CI 15.6%–47.4%).[35] That may indicate that the brain injury itself or confounders are also important for prognosis, which does of course not diminish the need for good and comprehensive epilepsy care (Table 3.5).

TABLE 3.4   Risk Factors of Pharmacoresistance[69]

Younger age
Status epilepticus
Epileptiform EEG abnormality
Focal onset seizure

TABLE 3.5   Clinical Take-Home Messages

- Post-traumatic epilepsy is more common after severe traumatic brain injury.
- There is no evidence that primary prophylaxis with antiseizure medication prevents epilepsy.
- A first unprovoked seizure >7 days after trauma indicates a higher risk (46%) than an acute symptomatic seizure. The risk is particularly high (≥75%) if it was a very severe traumatic brain injury.
- There are few studies comparing different ASMs in post-traumatic epilepsy.
- Cognitive problems and overrepresentation of psychosocial issues may complicate management, so a focus on compliance may be helpful.

REFERENCES

1. Pease M, Gupta K, Moshe SL, Correa DJ, Galanopoulou AS, Okonkwo DO, et al. Insights into epileptogenesis from post-traumatic epilepsy. Nat. Rev. Neurol. 2024 May;20:298–312.
2. Christensen J. The epidemiology of post-traumatic epilepsy. Semin. Neurol. 2015 June; 35:218–222.
3. Salazar AM, Schwab K, Grafman JH. Penetrating injuries in the Vietnam war: traumatic unconsciousness, epilepsy, and psychosocial outcome. Neurosurg. Clin. N. Am. 1995 October;6:715–726.
4. Kazemi H, Hashemi-Fesharaki S, Razaghi S, Najafi M, Kolivand PH, Kovac S, et al. Intractable epilepsy and craniocerebral trauma: analysis of 163 patients with blunt and penetrating head injuries sustained in war. Injury. 2012 December;43:2132–2135.
5. Syvertsen M, Nakken KO, Edland A, Hansen G, Hellum MK, Koht J. Prevalence and etiology of epilepsy in a Norwegian county —a population based study. Epilepsia. 2015 May;56:699–706.
6. Annegers JF, Hauser WA, Coan SP, Rocca WA. A population-based study of seizures after traumatic brain injuries. N. Engl. J. Med. 1998 January 1;338:20–24.
7. Karlander M, Ljungqvist J, Zelano J. Post-traumatic epilepsy in adults: a nationwide register-based study. J. Neurol. Neurosurg. Psychiatry. 2021 March 9;92:617–621.
8. Xu T, Yu X, Ou S, Liu X, Yuan J, Huang H, et al. Risk factors for post-traumatic epilepsy: a systematic review and meta-analysis. Epilepsy Behav. 2017 February;67:1–6.
9. Laaksonen J, Ponkilainen V, Kuitunen I, Mottonen J, Mattila VM. Association between pediatric traumatic brain injury and epilepsy at later ages in Finland: a nationwide register-based cohort study. Epilepsia. 2023 December;64:3257–3265.
10. Tubi MA, Lutkenhoff E, Blanco MB, McArthur D, Villablanca P, Ellingson B, et al. Early seizures and temporal lobe trauma predict post-traumatic epilepsy: a longitudinal study. Neurobiol. Dis. 2019 March;123:115–121.
11. Brady RD, Casillas-Espinosa PM, Agoston DV, Bertram EH, Kamnaksh A, Semple BD, et al. Modelling traumatic brain injury and post-traumatic epilepsy in rodents. Neurobiol. Dis. 2019 March;123:8–19.
12. Pitkanen A, Lukasiuk K. Mechanisms of epileptogenesis and potential treatment targets. Lancet Neurol. 2011 February;10:173–186.
13. Vespa PM, Shrestha V, Abend N, Agoston D, Au A, Bell MJ, et al. The epilepsy bioinformatics study for anti-epileptogenic therapy (EpiBioS4Rx) clinical biomarker: study design and protocol. Neurobiol. Dis. 2019 March;123:110–114.
14. Pease M, Elmer J, Shahabadi AZ, Mallela AN, Ruiz-Rodriguez JF, Sexton D, et al. Predicting post-traumatic epilepsy using admission electroencephalography after severe traumatic brain injury. Epilepsia. 2023 July;64:1842–1852.
15. Christensen J, Pedersen MG, Pedersen CB, Sidenius P, Olsen J, Vestergaard M. Long-term risk of epilepsy after traumatic brain injury in children and young adults: a population-based cohort study. Lancet. 2009 March 28;373:1105–1110.
16. Cotter D, Kelso A, Neligan A. Genetic biomarkers of post-traumatic epilepsy: a systematic review. Seizure. 2017 March;46:53–58.
17. Lolk K, Dreier JW, Christensen J. Repeated traumatic brain injury and risk of epilepsy: a Danish nationwide cohort study. Brain J. Neurol. 2021 April 12;144:875–884.
18. Christensen J, Pedersen HS, Fenger-Gron M, Fann JR, Jones NC, Vestergaard M. Selective serotonin reuptake inhibitors and risk of epilepsy after traumatic brain injury–a population based cohort study. PLOS ONE. 2019;14:e0219137.

19. Garner R, La Rocca M, Vespa P, Jones N, Monti MM, Toga AW, et al. Imaging biomarkers of post-traumatic epileptogenesis. Epilepsia. 2019 November;60:2151–2162.

20. Hlauschek G, Lossius MI, Schwartz DL, Silbert LC, Hicks AJ, Ponsford JL, et al. Reduced total number of enlarged perivascular spaces in post-traumatic epilepsy patients with unilateral lesions–a feasibility study. Seizure. 2023 December;113:1–5.

21. Pyrzowski J, Kalas M, Mazurkiewicz-Beldzinska M, Sieminski M. EEG biomarkers for the prediction of post-traumatic epilepsy–a systematic review of an emerging field. Seizure. 2024 July;119:71–77.

22. Eickholtz A, Abbas S, James E, Gibson C, Iskander G, Lypka M, et al. Ride the wave: continuous electroencephalography is indicated in the management of traumatic. Brain Injury Clin. EEG Neurosci. 2022 November;53:513–518.

23. Young B, Rapp RP, Norton JA, Haack D, Tibbs PA, Bean JR. Failure of prophylactically administered phenytoin to prevent late post-traumatic seizures. J. Neurosurg. 1983 February; 58:236–241.

24. Temkin NR, Dikmen SS, Wilensky AJ, Keihm J, Chabal S, Winn HR. A randomized, double-blind study of phenytoin for the prevention of post-traumatic seizures. N. Engl. J. Med. 1990 August 23;323:497–502.

25. Wilson CD, Burks JD, Rodgers RB, Evans RM, Bakare AA, Safavi-Abbasi S. Early and late post-traumatic epilepsy in the setting of traumatic brain injury: a meta-analysis and review of antiepileptic management. World Neurosurg. 2018 February;110:e901–e906.

26. Jennett B. Post-traumatic epilepsy: phenytoin prophylaxis. J. Neurosurg. 1980 February; 52:291.

27. Johnson AL, Harris P, McQueen JK, Blackwood DH, Kalbag RM. Phenytoin prophylaxis for post-traumatic seizures. J. Neurosurg. 1983 October;59:727–731.

28. Bakr A, Belli A. A systematic review of levetiracetam versus phenytoin in the prevention of late post-traumatic seizures and survey of UK neurosurgical prescribing practice of antiepileptic medication in acute traumatic brain injury. Br. J. Neurosurg. 2018 June;32:237–244.

29. Pearl PL, McCarter R, McGavin CL, Yu Y, Sandoval F, Trzcinski S, et al. Results of phase II levetiracetam trial following acute head injury in children at risk for post-traumatic epilepsy. Epilepsia. 2013 September;54:e135–e137.

30. Ferguson PL, Smith GM, Wannamaker BB, Thurman DJ, Pickelsimer EE, Selassie AW. A population-based study of risk of epilepsy after hospitalization for traumatic brain injury. Epilepsia. 2010 May;51:891–898.

31. Raymont V, Salazar AM, Lipsky R, Goldman D, Tasick G, Grafman J. Correlates of post-traumatic epilepsy 35 years following combat brain injury. Neurology. 2010 July 20;75:224–229.

32. Keret A, Bennett-Back O, Rosenthal G, Gilboa T, Shweiki M, Shoshan Y, et al. Post-traumatic epilepsy: long-term follow-up of children with mild traumatic brain injury. J. Neurosurg. Pediatr. 2017 July;20:64–70.

33. DeGrauw X, Thurman D, Xu L, Kancherla V, DeGrauw T. Epidemiology of traumatic brain injury-associated epilepsy and early use of anti-epilepsy drugs: an analysis of insurance claims data, 2004–2014. Epilepsy Res. 2018 October;146:41–49.

34. Chen Z, Laing J, Li J, O'Brien TJ, Gabbe BJ, Semple BD. Hospital-acquired infections as a risk factor for post-traumatic epilepsy: a registry-based cohort study. Epilepsia Open. 2024 May; 9(4):1333–1344.

35. Hesdorffer DC, Benn EK, Cascino GD, Hauser WA. Is a first acute symptomatic seizure epilepsy? Mortality and risk for recurrent seizure. Epilepsia. 2009 May;50:1102–1108.

36. Karlander M, Hakansson S, Ljungqvist J, Sorbo A, Zelano J. Risk of epilepsy following a first post-traumatic seizure: a register-based study. Neurol. Clin. Pract. 2025 February; 15:e200409.

37. Haltiner AM, Temkin NR, Dikmen SS. Risk of seizure recurrence after the first late post-traumatic seizure. Arch. Phys. Med. Rehabil. 1997 August;78:835–840.

38. Pease M, Gonzalez-Martinez J, Puccio A, Nwachuku E, Castellano JF, Okonkwo DO, et al. Risk factors and incidence of epilepsy after severe traumatic brain injury. Ann. Neurol. 2022 October;92:663–669.

39. Ritter AC, Wagner AK, Szaflarski JP, Brooks MM, Zafonte RD, Pugh MJ, et al. Prognostic models for predicting post-traumatic seizures during acute hospitalization, and at 1 and 2 years following traumatic brain injury. Epilepsia. 2016 September;57:1503–1514.

40. Won SY, Konczalla J, Dubinski D, Cattani A, Cuca C, Seifert V, et al. A systematic review of epileptic seizures in adults with subdural haematomas. Seizure. 2017 February;45: 28–35.

41. Spencer R, Manivannan S, Sharouf F, Bhatti MI, Zaben M. Risk factors for the development of seizures after cranioplasty in patients that sustained traumatic brain injury: a systematic review. Seizure. 2019 July;69:11–16.

42. Park JT, Chugani HT. Post-traumatic epilepsy in children-experience from a tertiary referral center. Pediatr. Neurol. 2015 February;52:174–181.

43. Kuhl NO, Yengo-Kahn AM, Burnette H, Solomon GS, Zuckerman SL. Sport-related concussive convulsions: a systematic review. Phys. Sportsmed. 2018 February;46:1–7.

44. Krumholz A, Wiebe S, Gronseth GS, Gloss DS, Sanchez AM, Kabir AA, et al. Evidence-based guideline: management of an unprovoked first seizure in adults: report of the Guideline Development Subcommittee of the American Academy of Neurology and the American Epilepsy Society. Neurology. 2015 April 21;84:1705–1713.

45. Lawn N, Chan J, Lee J, Dunne J. Is the first seizure epilepsy—and when? Epilepsia. 2015 September;56:1425–1431.

46. Zimmermann LL, Martin RM, Girgis F. Treatment options for post-traumatic epilepsy. Curr. Opin. Neurol. 2017 December;30:580–586.

47. Young B, Rapp RP, Norton JA, Haack D, Tibbs PA, Bean JR. Failure of prophylactically administered phenytoin to prevent early post-traumatic seizures. J. Neurosurg. 1983 February;58:231–235.

48. Young KD, Okada PJ, Sokolove PE, Palchak MJ, Panacek EA, Baren JM, et al. A randomized, double-blinded, placebo-controlled trial of phenytoin for the prevention of early post-traumatic seizures in children with moderate to severe blunt head injury. Ann. Emerg. Med. 2004 April;43:435–446.

49. Gopalan H, Krishnakumar P. Use of anti-epileptic drugs for post traumatic seizure: a global survey. Ann. Neurosci. 2023 January;30:26–32.

50. Gul N, Khan SA, Khattak HA, Muhammad G, Khan AA, Khan I, et al. Efficacy of phenytoin in prevention of early post-traumatic seizures. J. Ayub. Med. Coll. Abbottabad. 2019 April–June;31:237–241.

51. Generoso E, Diep C, Hua C, Rader E, Ran R, Lee NJ, et al. Assessing risk factors associated with breakthrough early post-traumatic seizures in patients receiving phenytoin prophylaxis. Front. Neurol. 2023;14:1329042.

52. Inaba K, Menaker J, Branco BC, Gooch J, Okoye OT, Herrold J, et al. A prospective multicenter comparison of levetiracetam versus phenytoin for early post-traumatic seizure prophylaxis. J. Trauma Acute Care Surg. 2013 March;74:766–771; discussion 771–763.

53. Glaser AC, Kanter JH, Martinez-Camblor P, Taenzer A, Anderson MV, Buhl L, et al. The effect of antiseizure medication administration on mortality and early post-traumatic seizures in critically ill older adults with traumatic brain injury. Neurocrit. Care. 2022 October;37:538–546.

54. Chaari A, Mohamed AS, Abdelhakim K, Kauts V, Casey WF. Levetiracetam versus phenytoin for seizure prophylaxis in brain injured patients: a systematic review and meta-analysis. Int. J. Clin. Pharm. 2017 October;39:998–1003.

55. Khan NR, VanLandingham MA, Fierst TM, Hymel C, Hoes K, Evans LT, et al. Should levetiracetam or phenytoin be used for post-traumatic seizure prophylaxis? a systematic review of the literature and meta-analysis. Neurosurgery. 2016 December;79:775–782.

56. Lee CH, Koo HW, Han SR, Choi CY, Sohn MJ, Lee CH. Phenytoin versus levetiracetam as prophylaxis for postcraniotomy seizure in patients with no history of seizures: systematic review and meta-analysis. J. Neurosurg. 2019 June 1;130:1–8.

57. Piccenna L, Shears G, O'Brien TJ. Management of post-traumatic epilepsy: an evidence review over the last 5 years and future directions. Epilepsia Open. 2017 June;2:123–144.

58. Wyllie E. Wyllie's treatment of epilepsy: principles and practice. 7th ed. Philadelphia: LWW; 2020.

59. Hakansson S, Karlander M, Larsson D, Mahamud Z, Garcia-Ptacek S, Zelezniak A, et al. Potential for improved retention rate by personalized antiseizure medication selection: a register-based analysis. Epilepsia. 2021 September;62:2123–2132.

60. Ferreira LD, Tabaeizadeh M, Haneef Z. Surgical outcomes in post-traumatic temporal lobe epilepsy: a systematic review and meta-analysis. J. Neurotrauma. 2024 February;41:319–330.

61. Kuo JR, Su BY. Neuropsychological impairments in patients with post-traumatic epilepsy: a scoping review. World Neurosurg. 2023 August;176:85–97.

62. Haltiner AM, Temkin NR, Winn HR, Dikmen SS. The impact of post-traumatic seizures on 1-year neuropsychological and psychosocial outcome of head injury. J. Int. Neuropsychol. Soc. 1996 November;2:494–504.

63. Foreman B, Lee H, Mizrahi MA, Hartings JA, Ngwenya LB, Privitera M, et al. Seizures and cognitive outcome after traumatic brain injury: a post hoc analysis. Neurocrit. Care. 2022 February;36:130–138.

64. Schneider ALC, Law CA, Gottesman RF, Krauss G, Huang J, Kucharska-Newton A, et al. Post-traumatic epilepsy and dementia risk. JAMA Neurol. 2024 February 26;81:346–353.

65. Gugger JJ, Kennedy E, Panahi S, Tate DF, Roghani A, Van Cott AC, et al. Multimodal quality of life assessment in post-9/11 veterans with epilepsy: impact of drug resistance, traumatic brain injury, and comorbidity. Neurology. 2022 April 26;98:e1761–e1770.

66. Juengst SB, Wagner AK, Ritter AC, Szaflarski JP, Walker WC, Zafonte RD, et al. Post-traumatic epilepsy associations with mental health outcomes in the first two years after moderate to severe TBI: a TBI model systems analysis. Epilepsy Behav. 2017 August;73:240–246.

67. Park KM, Shin KJ, Ha SY, Park J, Kim SE, Kim SE. Response to antiepileptic drugs in partial epilepsy with structural lesions on MRI. Clin. Neurol. Neurosurg. 2014 August;123:64–68.

68. Yu T, Liu X, Sun L, Wu J, Wang Q. Clinical characteristics of post-traumatic epilepsy and the factors affecting the latency of PTE. BMC Neurol. 2021 August 5;21:301.

69. Yu T, Liu X, Sun L, Lv R, Wu J, Wang Q. Risk factors for drug-resistant epilepsy (DRE) and a nomogram model to predict DRE development in post-traumatic epilepsy patients. CNS Neurosci. Ther. 2022 October;28:1557–1567.

70. Uski J, Lamusuo S, Teperi S, Loyttyniemi E, Tenovuo O. Mortality after traumatic brain injury and the effect of post-traumatic epilepsy. Neurology. 2018 August 28;91:e878–e883.

71. Lin WJ, Harnod T, Lin CL, Kao CH. Mortality risk and risk factors in patients with post-traumatic epilepsy: a population-based cohort study. Int. J. Environ. Res. Public Health. 2019 February 18;16:589.

72. Karlander M, Ljungqvist J, Sorbo A, Zelano J. Risk and cause of death in post-traumatic epilepsy: a register-based retrospective cohort study. J. Neurol. 2022 November;269:6014–6020.

73. Englander J, Bushnik T, Wright JM, Jamison L, Duong TT. Mortality in late post-traumatic seizures. J. Neurotrauma. 2009 September;26:1471–1477.

74. Sveinsson O, Andersson T, Carlsson S, Tomson T. Type, etiology, and duration of epilepsy as risk factors for SUDEP: further analyses of a population-based case-control study. Neurology. 2023 November 27;101:e2257–e2265.

Epilepsy after Brain Infections

4

4.1 RISK OF EPILEPSY

CNS infections are the most common preventable cause of epilepsy worldwide and explain a large portion of the difference in epilepsy prevalence between high- and low-middle-income countries.[1,2] Although risks and pathogens vary with geography, infections are important to consider as an epilepsy etiology in all parts of the world. With increased global mobility, there is a need for broader clinical vigilance in more countries to avoid diagnostic delay of treatable causes like neurocysticercosis and tuberculosis.[3] The most common infections causing epilepsy are viral encephalitis, abscesses, neurocysticercosis, and tuberculosis, but any brain infection like bacterial meningitis or opportunistic infections in the setting of immunocompromise may in rarer circumstances have the same result. From a societal perspective, vaccinations, other preventive measures, and improved treatment of infections are important tools in decreasing postinfectious epilepsy.

4.1.1 Prevalence

In developed countries, only a few percent of patients seen in epilepsy clinics have postinfectious epilepsy. For example in tertiary epilepsy centers in France, epilepsy of infectious etiology accounted for only 6% of cases.[4] This contrasts with higher rates (up to 20%–25%) in some low- and middle-income countries.[3] Importantly, prevalence of epilepsy of infectious causes is difficult to estimate for various reasons. Attribution of epilepsy to an infectious etiology may be more common in areas with higher rates of likely culprit infections. Several infections, like tuberculosis, viral encephalitis, and neurocysticercosis, may cause acute symptomatic seizures rather than epilepsy, but the distinction may not be noticed in routine follow-up outside epilepsy care providers. That patients with acute symptomatic seizures are diagnosed with epilepsy may inflate prevalence estimates.

4.1.2 Incidence

The epilepsy risk after a CNS infection varies with the pathogen and severity of residual lesions but is overall probably a few percent in most industrialized countries.[3] In the USA, Annegers and colleagues described a 7% survival-adjusted risk in the 20 years following encephalitis or meningitis, with the highest risk seen in the first years.[5] Similarly, the 10-year risk was 6% in adult patients hospitalized for CNS infections in Sweden between 2000 and 2010 (Figure 4.1).[6] These results contrasts to the developing world, where rates after CNS infections range from 12% to 25% or higher, depending on the panorama of infectious agents.[3]

A difficulty in determining the risk of epilepsy after brain infections lies in the relatively long follow-up needed and how much of later epilepsy is attributed to brain infections in childhood. For instance, some patients undergoing surgery for mesial temporal lobe sclerosis have had a childhood brain infection, but causal associations are difficult to establish and the risk of recall bias is probably substantial.[3] Similarly, neurocysticercosis is a common infection in some areas but does not invariably cause epilepsy, which raises the risk of misattribution of later epilepsy.

4.1.3 Risks after Particular Infections

4.1.3.1 Herpes Virus Encephalitis

Herpes simplex virus (HSV) encephalitis is the most common sporadic encephalitis and often caused by HSV-1, but HSV-2 accounts for a proportion of cases, particularly in the immunocompromised. It is one of the most common causes of postviral epilepsy, and about one fourth of survivors seem to develop epilepsy.[7,8] Acute symptomatic seizures

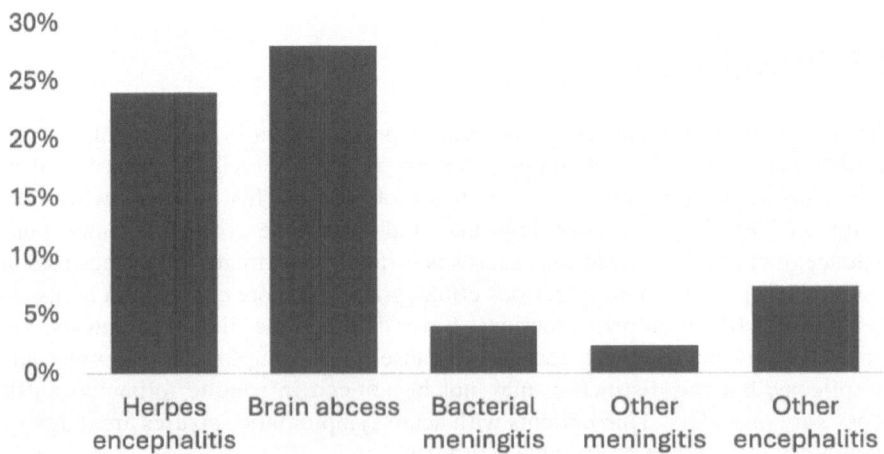

FIGURE 4.1   Ten-year cumulative incidence of epilepsy after different brain infections in Sweden 2000–2010.

may occur in up to 40%–60% of cases.[9] MRI changes are associated with epilepsy, so presumably many cases of epilepsy result from brain lesions or structural changes caused by the infection.[7] Among 45 patients at the Mayo Clinic (HSV-1 in 33 and HSV-2 in 9), seizures were a presenting symptom in 18%, and six patients (13%) had status epilepticus. At last follow-up, 10 patients (46% of those for which data were available) had epilepsy.[10] In population-based investigations in Sweden, 24% of survivors of verified HSV encephalitis in 1990–2001 were readmitted for epilepsy after a median of nine months.[11] A subsequent study found that the 10-year risk of epilepsy was similar for adults in Sweden hospitalized with HSV encephalitis in 2000–2010, about 26%.[6]

4.1.3.2 Other Viral Encephalitides

Many viruses can result in encephalitis, but because of geographic variability and since the specific virus is frequently not identified, there are relatively few population-based investigations.[9] HSV is most the common cause of sporadic cases, but encephalitis can also be caused by influenzas, measles, mumps, enteroviruses, varizella zoster virus (VZV), and West Nile virus, to name a few.[7] The epilepsy risk is influenced by the different anatomical predilection of different viruses for different brain areas. Herpes virus and Japanese encephalitis both increase the risk of epilepsy compared to encephalitis of other causes.[12] However, HSV-1 has affinity for basal-frontal and temporal cortex,[9] which results in higher epilepsy rates than Japanese encephalitis, which has a subcortical predilection.[3] In a study from Taiwan, epilepsy developed in 16%–26% of children with acute encephalitis, out of which 80% of those with epilepsy had their first seizure within six months.[12,13] Risk factors for epilepsy were acute symptomatic seizures, status epilepticus, disturbed level of consciousness, focal neurological signs, abnormal EEG, and focal abnormalities on imaging. Children with acute symptomatic seizures had a five-year risk of epilepsy of 33%, compared to 1.2% in children without any seizure during the index admission. Among children infected with the chikungunya virus in Honduras and admitted for neurological symptoms, 10% had seizures.[14]

Cytomegalovirus (CMV) can cause severe encephalitis, mainly after transplantation. A case report describes postencephalitic epilepsy four years after CMV encephalitis at two months of age, with excellent response to carbamazepine—but the epilepsy may have been coincidental.[15]

4.1.3.3 Bacterial Meningitis

Epilepsy after bacterial meningitis is rarer than after viral encephalitis. In case series, about 15%–20% seem to have acute symptomatic seizures, which are associated with focal imaging findings and severe disease.[16] Long-term risks are around a few percent in most studies, both in adults and children.[3,17,18] The 10-year risk was 4% in adult patients hospitalized for bacterial meningitis and surviving the acute phase in Sweden in 2000–2010.[6] Longer-term risks of epilepsy are difficult to assess, since bacterial meningitis is sometimes considered a risk factor for subsequent mesial temporal lobe epilepsy.[3,19]

4.1.3.4 Brain Abscesses

Acute symptomatic seizures occur in a quarter of patients with brain abscesses, and many will develop subsequent epilepsy that can be drug resistant.[17] The 10-year risk of epilepsy was 30% (95% CI 27%–33%) in survivors of a brain abscess in Sweden in 2000–2010, which is very similar to results from Demark.[6,20] An early single-center series reported epilepsy in about the same proportion, but a more recent series did not.[21,22] In the latter series, only 7% of patients developed epilepsy.[22] Differences in inclusion criteria may account for some of the difference. Epilepsy most often develops in the first few years after the abscess diagnosis.[22] Risk factors for epilepsy are seizures during admission for brain abscess, neurosurgery, alcoholism, frontal lobe abscess, and stroke.[23]

4.1.3.5 Syphilis

Neurosyphilis was once common but is now less so in developed countries. Most studies are small and single center. A study from Bangalore, India, reported that out of 119 patients with neurosyphilis with a median age of 38 at diagnosis, 30 patients (25%) had seizures at some point during the disease course. Tonic-clonic seizures were seen in 17 patients and focal seizures in eight. Seizures were reportedly controlled in 25 patients in the acute phase, but long-term data on epilepsy and drug response were not reported.[24]

4.1.3.6 Tuberculosis

Tuberculosis (TB) is a common infection in developing countries and can cause epilepsy through meningitis (TBM), tuberculomas, or associated stroke.[25] A study in India reported seizures in 27 (34%) of 79 mainly adult patients with TBM between 2014 and 2019, and most occurred prior to hospitalization.[26] Focal onset seizures were the most common type. Seizures were attributed to meningeal irritation, tuberculoma irritating the cortex, or vascular pathology. Hyponatremia was also found to be an independent risk factor for seizures.[26] Reported risks of epilepsy vary substantially, perhaps because of care administered and age of the studied cohorts. A study of 40 children with TBM in Pakistan reported epilepsy in 76% of survivors.[27] In Auckland, 29 out of 104 patients with TBM (28%) had seizures during the hospitalization, but only nine out of 81 survivors (11%) developed epilepsy.[28] Notably, 33% had stroke as a complication to their tuberculosis. Antitubercular treatment can in itself cause seizures, which complicates interpretation of the literature.[25]

4.1.3.7 Neurocysticercosis

Neurocysticercosis is caused by the tapeworm *Tannia solium* and believed to cause a substantial proportion of epilepsy cases in certain areas of the world.[3] In Namibia, 51% of 177 patients with new-onset seizures and a mean age of 31 had suspected neurocysticercosis on neuroimaging.[29] Importantly, many of the seizures that occur during the immunological reaction to the cysts are probably acute symptomatic and patients may not develop epilepsy (an enduring predisposition for seizures after treatment).[30] Pathogenic mechanisms can include edema, gliosis, and the immune-response to cysts in different forms.[17] MRI is required, and differential diagnoses include toxoplasmosis, metastases, and tuberculomas.[3] The epilepsy does not seem particularly difficult to treat, but studies are lacking and rates of actual drug resistance difficult to obtain.

4.1.3.8 HIV

HIV is reported to cause epilepsy and seizures, but much of the literature probably reflects a previous treatment era with regards to the infection. If epilepsy is encountered in the setting of HIV, important management considerations include interactions between ASM and antiretroviral medications. Modern HIV treatment has made neurological sequelae rarer in countries with modern health care. If the virus is not controlled, approximately 20% of all patents with HIV-associated neurological symptoms develop seizures.[31] Etiologies include opportunistic infections as well as metabolic disturbances. Toxoplasmosis, cryptococcal meningitis, and tuberculosis may cause epilepsy in HIV-positive individuals, as may lymphoma and progressive multifocal leukoencephalopathy.[31] A South African retrospective study of children with HIV infection in 2008–2015 found that 23% had a history of seizures, but the local panorama of CNS infections was likely of importance, since prior bacterial meningitis and tuberculosis were significant risk factors. Another risk factor was cerebrovascular events—perhaps caused by HIV-associated vascular disease. Two thirds of the children with seizures were diagnosed with epilepsy. A total of 33% of the children did not have one year of seizure freedom, and valproic acid was the most commonly used ASM.[32]

4.1.3.9 Other Infections

Cryptococcal meningitis can be associated with HIV or other immunosuppressed situations. In a series of HIV-negative cases, 28 out of 180 patients had seizures—13 acute symptomatic and 15 late seizures, after a mean interval of 1.5 and 51.4 days, respectively.[33] Two out of 13 survivors (15%) had drug-resistant epilepsy.[33]

Neurobrucellosis is a zoonotic disease transmitted through underprocessed food, relatively more common around the Mediterranean Sea. Epilepsy may complicate meningoencephalitis, particularly if intracerebral granulomas are present.[34]

Other parasitic CNS infection also cause epilepsy. A problem with the epidemiology of parasitic causes of epilepsy is that patients may not undergo neuroimaging in countries where parasites are common, and the etiology of epilepsy simply be inferred from serological evidence or history congruent with previous infection.[17] One clear example is cerebral malaria, which can cause acute encephalopathy with seizures but also increase the risk of subsequent epilepsy. Whether this is most often a result of the infection itself or associated vasculopathy and stroke is unknown.[17]

4.2 EPILEPTOGENESIS

The mechanisms of epileptogenesis in most infectious epilepsies have been suggested to include structural changes, immune changes, blood–brain barrier disruption, gliosis, synaptic reorganization, and epigenetic mechanisms.[17] The acute inflammatory response may cause acute symptomatic seizures, and longer-lasting immune mechanisms are potentially involved in epileptogenesis.[35] These could be both pathogen-mediated and host response-mediated effects, with ensuing inflammation and network changes leading to epilepsy.[17]

Temporally, infectious epilepsy follows a pattern resembling that seen after other brain insults, suggesting that general mechanisms of epileptogenesis are at work. After brain infections in adults, epilepsy typically arises in the first two years, but the risk remains slightly above normal for an extended period of time beyond that phase.[6] Together with the fact that acute symptomatic seizures are a clear risk factor for later epilepsy, it seems that epileptogenesis at least temporally resembles that seen after stroke or traumatic brain injury.

Some specific mechanisms have been linked to distinct etiologies; the immune response to HSV is able to trigger an autoimmune response through antibody formation caused by similarities between peptides in the virus and synaptic proteins.[35] This can cause autoimmune encephalitis in close temporal proximity (usually weeks) to HSV encephalitis, resulting in a biphasic clinical course. In addition, there is the concept of brain infections in childhood resulting in later mesial temporal lobe sclerosis, a theory that reflects the overrepresentation of an early childhood infection in surgical series. Demonstrating causality over such extended periods of times is difficult, but a recent meta-analysis found that HHV-6 DNA is more commonly detected than by chance in patients that have undergone surgery for temporal lobe epilepsy.[9,17,36]

Specific pathophysiological mechanisms are also suggested for neurocysticercosis, including edema around the cysts, the immunological response, calcification of the cysts, and tissue damage caused by the infection.[30,37] Blood–brain barrier dysfunction is also suggested to be involved, since host immune response against the infection results in altered permeability and access of peripheral inflammation to the CNS. Seizures often start to occur at the time a cyst degenerates, which coincides with pericystical edema on imaging. So far, anti-inflammatory treatment does not seem to reduce the risk of epilepsy, and there are concerns that excessive immunotherapy may compromise the immunological checks that keep the infection suppressed.[37] Similar mechanisms have been suggested for tuberculosis and brain abcesses.[25]

Antiepileptogenesis treatment consists mainly of treating the infection, and there have been no recent studies reported on antiseizure medications used as prophylaxis in neurocysticercosis.[38] In tuberculosis, abscesses, or encephalitides, the relevant anti-infectious treatment is usually combined with steroids to reduce the inflammatory response, but protocols vary and are beyond the scope of this book.

4.3 RISK FACTORS

The main risk factors for epilepsy after brain infection seem to be acute symptomatic seizures,[5] including status epilepticus during the acute phase, parenchymal brain lesions, severe disease requiring intensive care, and particular infections (Table 4.1).[3] Children seem to have a somewhat higher risk of postinfectious epilepsy than adults, but whether this represents age differences in epileptogenic potential, panorama of infections, outcomes, or longer follow-up is difficult to determine.[3]

Acute symptomatic seizures occur during the active phase of the infection. Risk factors are usually a severe infection, cortical location of lesions, and epileptiform discharges on EEG.[39] In a Korean study, 23% of all patients with CNS infections exhibited acute symptomatic seizures, with encephalitis and neurological deficits being risk factors.[40]

Risk factors of epilepsy after a viral encephalitis mimic those of all infections and include reduced level of consciousness, early seizure, status epilepticus, MRI abnormality, EEG abnormality, and positive herpes simplex virus in cerebrospinal fluid.[41] In contrast to the instant brain insults due to stroke or traumatic brain injury, in which acute symptomatic seizures usually occur in the first day, seizures in brain infections can arise also a few days after diagnosis. For instance, the average time to onset of acute symptomatic seizures in a series of brain abscesses was 2.3 days.[22]

4.4 RISK OF EPILEPSY AFTER A FIRST SEIZURE

Conceptually, the distinction between seizures occurring in the acute phase and seizures occurring later is the same in brain infections as in all other brain diseases. The insidious onset of infections and the long duration of the insult makes it harder to correctly determine when the acute symptomatic phase has ended. If there is an active infection with ongoing brain stress, the acute symptomatic phase may probably extend beyond a week. To take this problem into account, early seizures have often been defined as seizures occurring in the two weeks after brain infections.[3,17] Clinically, it is more important to determine if a seizure occurred during the time of an active brain infection rather than ascertaining the exact timing in relation to the first infectious symptom.

TABLE 4.1   Risk Factors of Epilepsy after Brain Infection

Early seizures
Severe infection (requiring intensive care)
Parenchymal lesions
Infection type
Age

4.4.1 Risk of Seizure Recurrence after an Acute Symptomatic Seizure

Regarding the risk of seizure recurrence, Hesdorffer and colleagues found a risk of an unprovoked seizure after a first acute symptomatic seizure of 16.6% (95% CI = 9.5%–28.0%) in the US in 1955–1984.[42] The confidence interval was wide because of low participant numbers, and the population was mainly pediatric. In a more recent Korean study, 14/34 patients (41%) developed epilepsy after a first acute symptomatic seizure.[40] In encephalitis, status epilepticus as an acute symptomatic seizure is not uncommon and may indicate a greater risk of later unprovoked seizures.[3]

Seizure during the acute phase of the infection seems to be a risk factor for later epilepsy, but just like in some immune-mediated epilepsies it may be difficult to determine when the acute symptomatic phase ends. On illustrative case series on neurocysticercosis describes that only 13 patients out of over 50 with a first seizure developed recurrent seizures,[43] indicating that treatment of the infection might have prevented actual epileptogenesis and that the first seizures had been acute symptomatic.

4.4.2 Risk of Seizure Recurrence after an Unprovoked Seizure

Most studies describing recurrence risks in CNS infections have either very short follow-up or few adult patients. In Minnesota in 1955–1984, the risk of an unprovoked seizure after a first late seizure occurring more than one week after the infection was 63.5% (95% CI = 21.2%–98.6%), but the population was small and of mixed ages, resulting in the very wide confidence interval.[42]

As in other acquired epilepsies, it is likely that the presence of general risk factors (focal lesion, large lesion, acute symptomatic seizure) can inform the assessment of risk of subsequent seizures. A higher recurrence risk could motivate ASM treatment already after one seizure in some patients. What pathogen-stratified data exist supports this notion: reported risks of seizure recurrence in specific etiologies are 30%–65% for HIV[44–46] and 18%–33% for neurocysticercosis,[43,47,48] but for brain abscesses, recurrence rates are reported up to 81%,[21] although later studies reported lower rates, which can perhaps reflect either differences in definition of brain abscesses or advances in the acute care of them.[22] The first two etiologies are very clinically heterogeneous and ascertainment may only have been by serology, in contrast to brain abscesses where there is a focal lesion. Strangely, there is no robust data concerning recurrence risks after first seizures after HSV encephalitis, a common cause of infectious epilepsy.[9]

There could also be age differences in recurrence risks. Some pediatric articles on bacterial meningitis suggest high seizure recurrence risks, but the studies are also relatively old.[5,49,50] There are some more recent large population-based studies describing seizures in or after brain infections, but they combine acute symptomatic and unprovoked seizures and do not report recurrence risks after just one remote seizure, which is the interesting question when a patient has had a single seizure.[7,11,51–53]

There is currently no data on the importance of latency from the infection to the first seizure in assessment of recurrence risk, but after other brain lesions epilepsy typically arises in the first few years.

4.5 MANAGEMENT

4.5.1 Clinical Presentation

Epilepsy in brain infections presents in different clinical settings. For acute symptomatic seizures, there is usually but not always the context of an acute febrile infection. Prodromal symptoms like headache or remote symptoms from ear-nose-throat or cough can give clues. In cases of encephalitis there may be strange behaviors or hallucinations before the onset. In all cases of altered level of consciousness or suspicion of non-convulsive or subtle status epilepticus, cerebral infection should be on the list of differentials diagnoses. Similarly, infectious causes need to be ruled out early by imaging and CSF examination in most guidelines regarding status epilepticus. One needs to follow local treatment and investigation protocols.

Status epilepticus is probably not an uncommon presentation of acute brain infection, but the proportion varies with setting and age. Infectious or immunological etiology accounted for at least a quarter of status epilepticus cases in a pediatric cohort of new-onset refractory status epilepticus (NORSE) studied in South Korea.[54] In contrast, only eight out of over 200 (<4%) cases of status epilepticus in Salzburg, Austria, had infectious or immune-mediated etiology of their status epilepticus.[55]

Both focal and bilateral tonic-clonic seizures have been reported in the acute symptomatic phase. For example, in a series with tuberculosis, focal seizures occurred in 14%, focal to bilateral tonic-clonic 11%, tonic-clonic at onset 9%, and status epilepticus in 8%.[26] Similarly, a very wide range of seizure types, from focal motor and bilateral tonic-clonic seizures to myoclonic ones, have been reported in brain abscesses or bacterial meningitis.[22,56]

4.5.1.1 Presentation after the Infection

In the non-acute setting, suspicion that an epilepsy is the result of an infection can arise either because of a history of a treated CNS infection or because radiological findings in the work-up of a first seizure suggest an infectious cause. In the latter case, parenchymal lesions or meningeal alterations are examples that may give radiological suspicion of neurocysticercosis or tuberculosis. Infections disease consult is often required. Primary brain tumors, carcinomatosis, or other neoplasms like lymphoma as well as systemic inflammatory conditions can be important differential diagnoses. Repeat imaging and CSF examination are often helpful.

If there is a previously treated CNS infection and a first seizure arises after a typical latency, often in the first or second year, the case is more straightforward. The semiology of postinfectious epilepsy includes focal seizures with or without impaired awareness as well as bilateral tonic-clonic seizures. The exact symptoms depend on affected brain areas, but the semiology can be quite complex, particularly after viral encephalitis. For instance, a case series of postencephalitic epilepsy described complex sensory auras including auditory phenomenon.[57]

4.5.2 Estimating Recurrence Risk

When seeing a patient with a first seizure and a previous brain infection, estimating recurrence risk is important for good management (Figure 4.2). For many patients there will be evidence that the recurrence risk is higher than in unprovoked first seizures, but it will not be elevated sufficiently to motivate an epilepsy diagnosis according to the current ILAE definition. For many infections the risk is simply not known. Importantly, the decision about ASM treatment is separate from the epilepsy diagnosis. In cases of high recurrence risk (see earlier)—for instance in cases of cortical lesions after the infection and a typical latency of less than two years after the infection, or early seizures—patients may wish treatment and shared decision-making is essential, just like in other patients with an undetermined but probably elevated recurrence risk. One category that merits further study is brain abscesses, since as discussed previously, at least one early study reported a very high recurrence risk after a first unprovoked seizure.[21]

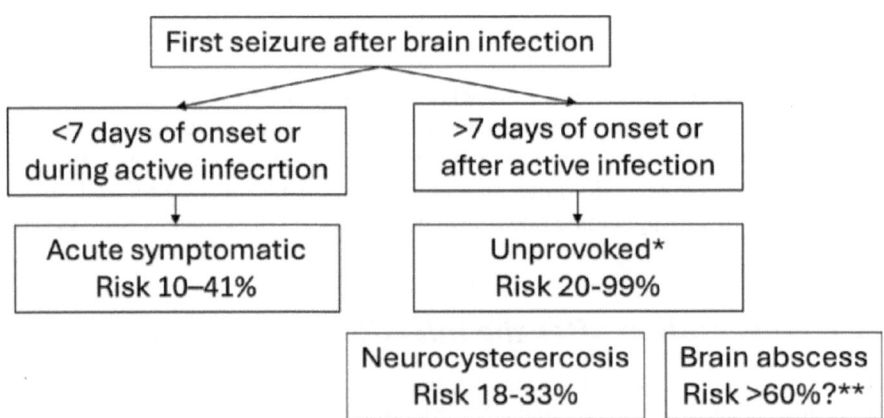

FIGURE 4.2   Risk of epilepsy after first seizures in different clinical situations.

Notes: * The very wide interval indicates the lack of studies. The risk is probably higher if there is parenchymal damage after the infection. ** The high risk after brain abscesses is from an early case series.

4.5.3 Treatment of Acute Symptomatic Seizures

Treatment of the infection is paramount to mitigate any direct and/or indirect CNS injury. Whether prompt treatment of meningitis or encephalitis with antimicrobial treatment or steroids reduces the risk of subsequent epilepsy is unknown, but treatment of parasites has been shown to be beneficial regarding the risk of epilepsy.[1,58] The most beneficial empiric antiviral and/or antibacterial treatment in each case depends on the local endemic infections.[1] Prompt treatment, neuroimaging, and blood and CSF examinations are most often needed.

Intravenous ASM administration is needed in cases of status epilepticus. In principle, ASMs without interactions may be preferable, but which drugs are available may also vary in different healthcare systems. Status epilepticus should be treated according to local guidelines. An important clinical course is NMDA-receptor encephalitis after HSV encephalitis, which emerges within weeks after HSV-1 infection. This can seem like a relapse but may require immunotherapy.[3] Regarding which ASM to use for acute symptomatic seizures, management considerations include patient comorbidities and potential for interactions with antimicrobial therapy.

4.5.4 Treatment of Epilepsy

The general considerations in ASM selection apply also for patients with epilepsy after a CNS infection. A good ASM is tolerable and prevents seizures, without interacting with other medications that the patient might need. There are relatively few studies describing longitudinal response to ASM treatment in postinfectious epilepsy.[1,58]

4.5.4.1 ASMs Specifically Studied in Infectious Epilepsy

There are not many studies providing high level evidence on ASM efficacy in the more common infectious etiologies like viral encephalitis, bacterial meningitis, and brain

TABLE 4.2 Selected RCTs on ASMs Evaluated in Acute Infections

STUDY	MAIN RESULT
ENCEPHALITIS	
Sharawat 2024[59]	Similar effect with regards to seizures in children with acute encephalitis (majority of infectious etiology) with phenytoin ($n = 50$) and levetiracetam ($n = 50$). More adverse effects with levetiracetam.
CEREBRAL MALARIA	
Birbeck 2019[60]	No difference between IV levetiracetam and IV phenobarbital with regards to seizures, coma duration, neurologic sequelae, or death, but levetiracetam was safer. Phenobarbital was discontinued in 3/15 cases due to respiratory side effects.

abscesses (Table 4.2). There are small studies and case series for other infections, particularly neurocysticercosis and tuberculosis, which overall convey the impression that most ASMs registered for focal epilepsy can probably be used and should be tailored to patient characteristics. In neurocysticercosis, one randomized trial compared levetiracetam and carbamazepine without finding any major significant differences in the effect on seizures.[61] A retrospective investigation of pediatric cases with the same infection found lacosamide to be approximately as effective as oxcarbazepine.[62] In a case series on epilepsy in tuberculosis describing ASM treatment, patients were most often treated with levetiracetam, and in one case valproate. Five patients required two ASMs, specifically levetiracetam and clobazam.[26]

4.5.5 Withdrawal

There is a scarcity of specific studies on withdrawal of ASMs in seizure-free patients with postinfectious epilepsy, so general guidelines must apply. Brain lesion, focal seizures, many seizures before remission, and short duration of seizure freedom are some risk factors for recurrence.[63] In some cases of infectious epilepsy, a patient may have ASM treatment because of seizures caused by an infection that was treated many years ago and it is unclear if epilepsy has actually developed or the seizures were acute symptomatic at the time. How long to continue such treatment is not known; clinical judgment and patient involvement are both important. After neurocysticercosis, studies have addressed the suitable length of ASM prophylaxis but have been inconclusive. Calcified lesions were suggested in one study to indicate a higher risk of epilepsy; if this holds true in future studies it may motivate longer treatment.[38] Importantly, there is an ongoing discussion that several patients with epilepsy in neurocysticercosis may in fact only have had acute symptomatic seizures, in which case epilepsy has not developed.[30] More research is needed.

4.5.6 Surgery

Epilepsy surgery may be underutilized in patients with infectious epilepsy, particularly since focal imaging abnormalities are more common in drug-resistant cases.[3,64] The high proportion of pharmacoresistance in infectious epilepsy and underrepresentation in epilepsy surgery series have been suggested to indicate too low rates of referral.[3] Case series describe successful outcomes of surgery for focal epilepsy post-HSV encephalitis, but just like for TB and presumably other CNS infections, there is a concern of reactivation of the original infection. In HSV reactivation, the first clinical sign seems to be fever followed by seizures.[3] Acyclovir prophylaxis during surgery has been described in case series.[65]

Since infectious etiologies are so rare in surgical case series, determining factors associated with good outcome is difficult. Temporal lobe surgery seems to be the most common resective surgery used in postinfectious epilepsy, but extratemporal surgery cases exist. In children with very large hemispheric damage after encephalitis, hemispherectomy is sometimes endeavored.[3] The literature contains a few cases of attempts at epilepsy surgery after bacterial meningitis; in these cases there was residual cortical scarring after presumed menigoencephalits.[3] As in all epilepsy surgery, individualized management and shared decision-making is key. There are case series describing beneficial effects of vagus nerve stimulation (VNS) in postencephalitic epilepsy, but the level of evidence is low.[66,67]

4.6 PROGNOSIS

4.6.1 Seizures

The literature contains many examples of high rates of drug-resistant epilepsy after brain infections.[3,64,68] In a large French multi-center cross-sectional study of epilepsy centers, approximately 40% of patients with epilepsy of infectious cause were seizure free with ASM treatment, 20% were not seizure free but still considered responders to ASM treatment, and 40% were non-responders.[4] After Japanese encephalitis, 78% of one series had continued seizures despite ASM treatment.[69]

The risk of medically refractory epilepsy seems to vary with etiology and severity of the initial injury (Table 4.3). This mimics other acquired epilepsies in which acute symptomatic seizures—reflecting a severe acute condition as well as cortical affliction—are a main risk factor. The risk seems highest after HSV encephalitis. In contrast, the epilepsy in neurocysticercosis is typically described as controllable, but whether this reflects poor follow-up or perhaps misclassification of acute symptomatic non-recurring seizures as epilepsy is difficult to know. Neurocysticercosis in children seems to have a lower risk of becoming medically refractory compared to adults, perhaps because of fewer calcified lesions.[3] Status epilepticus has also been reported as a risk factor for pharmacoresistance.[40] Other such factors include imaging abnormalities of temporal lobe structures and HSV infection.[3] In another investigation of infectious encephalitis, status epilepticus, focal seizures, intensive care, requiring several ASMs in the acute stage, imaging abnormalities, and epileptiform discharges on EEG were associated with later pharmacoresistance—but only status epilepticus was an independent predictor.[3]

TABLE 4.3 Risk Factors of Pharmacoresistance

Status epilepticus
Focal seizures
Severity of acute infection
Difficult-to-treat acute symptomatic seizures
Imaging abnormalities
Epileptiform discharges on EEG

4.6.2 Quality of Life

There are a few studies on quality of life in patients with epilepsy after brain infections. Overall, they echo findings in other remote symptomatic epilepsies and demonstrate the importance of seizure control as well as psychiatric comorbidities. In a study on 48 patients with neurocysticercosis and epilepsy, quality of life was reported as lower by patients with poor seizure control and depression compared to patients with neurocysticercosis but not epilepsy.[70] The most affected domains were social/family life and emotional well-being. Another study found the number of seizures to be the most important determinant of quality of life in neurocysticercosis.[71] Tonic-clonic seizures were mainly associated with lower quality of life scores. In other infectious etiologies, seizures are often considered an outcome next to quality of life, and there is a scarcity of studies examining associations between these.[72]

4.6.3 Mortality

Symptomatic epilepsy in general doubles mortality compared to persons with the same brain disorder that did not develop epilepsy. A composite estimate of the impact of all infectious epilepsy on the risk of death has not been reported and would be difficult to interpret. After all, different brain infections arise in very different settings. What information exists argues that the prognosis for survivors of brain infections with epilepsy could be better than for survivors of stroke or traumatic brain injury with epilepsy. A population-based follow-up study in Denmark found seizures to be a risk factor for both in-hospital mortality and later unfavorable outcome.[51] The impact of seizures on risk of mortality after the hospital admission was however considerably lower than for in-hospital mortality. A similar pattern was recently described for patients with brain abscess in Denmark. Epilepsy increased the risk of death during follow-up by approximately 25%,[23] which is considerably lower than the at least two-fold increased mortality normally associated with symptomatic epilepsy (Table 4.4).[73]

TABLE 4.4   Clinical Take-Home Messages

- Epilepsy after brain infection varies with geography, but travel increases the need for clinical vigilance worldwide.
- Herpes virus encephalitis, brain abscess, neurocysticercosis, and tuberculosis are common causes of epilepsy after brain infections.
- Etiological estimates are often uncertain, since lack of resources may prevent detection of alternative explanations for epilepsy.
- Early seizures occurring during the active infection have lower recurrence risk than later unprovoked seizures.
- Several common ASMs used in focal epilepsy have been reported in case series of postinfectious epilepsy, but the level of evidence is low.

REFERENCES

1. Singhi P. Infectious causes of seizures and epilepsy in the developing world. Dev. Med. Child. Neurol. 2011 July;53:600–609.
2. Feigin VL, Abajobir AA, Abate KH, Abd-Allah F, Abdulle AM, Abera SF, et al. Global, regional, and national burden of neurological disorders during 1990 –2015: a systematic analysis for the Global Burden of Disease Study 2015. Lancet Neurol. 2017;16:877–897.
3. Ramantani G, Holthausen H. Epilepsy after cerebral infection: review of the literature and the potential for surgery. Epileptic. Disord. 2017 June 1;19:117–136.
4. Chipaux M, Szurhaj W, Vercueil L, Milh M, Villeneuve N, Cances C, et al. Epilepsy diagnostic and treatment needs identified with a collaborative database involving tertiary centers in France. Epilepsia. 2016 May;57:757–769.
5. Annegers JF, Hauser WA, Beghi E, Nicolosi A, Kurland LT. The risk of unprovoked seizures after encephalitis and meningitis. Neurology. 1988 September;38:1407–1410.
6. Zelano J, Westman G. Epilepsy after brain infection in adults: a register-based population-wide study. Neurology. 2020 December 15;95:e3213–e3220.
7. Singh TD, Fugate JE, Hocker SE, Rabinstein AA. Postencephalitic epilepsy: clinical characteristics and predictors. Epilepsia. 2015 January;56:133–138.
8. Rocha ND, de Moura SK, da Silva GAB, Mattiello R, Sato DK. Neurological sequelae after encephalitis associated with herpes simplex virus in children: systematic review and meta-analysis. BMC Infect. Dis. 2023 January 26;23:55.
9. Misra UK, Tan CT, Kalita J. Viral encephalitis and epilepsy. Epilepsia. 2008 August;49 Suppl 6:13–18.
10. Singh TD, Fugate JE, Hocker S, Wijdicks EFM, Aksamit AJ Jr, Rabinstein AA. Predictors of outcome in HSV encephalitis. J. Neurol. 2016 February;263:277–289.
11. Hjalmarsson A, Blomqvist P, Skoldenberg B. Herpes simplex encephalitis in Sweden, 1990–2001: incidence, morbidity, and mortality. Clin. Infect. Dis. 2007 October 1;45:875–880.
12. Lee WT, Yu TW, Chang WC, Shau WY. Risk factors for postencephalitic epilepsy in children: a hospital-based study in Taiwan. Eur. J. Paediatr. Neurol. 2007 September;11:302–309.
13. Lin KL, Lin JJ, Hsia SH, Chou ML, Hung PC, Wang HS, et al. Effect of antiepileptic drugs for acute and chronic seizures in children with encephalitis. PLOS ONE. 2015;10:e0139974.
14. Samra JA, Hagood NL, Summer A, Medina MT, Holden KR. Clinical features and neurologic complications of children hospitalized with chikungunya virus in Honduras. J. Child. Neurol. 2017 July;32:712–716.
15. Nasuno M, Shigemura T, Nakazawa Y, Inaba Y, Motobayashi M. Postencephalitic epilepsy secondary to cytomegalovirus encephalitis. Pediatr. Int. 2018 August;60:758–760.
16. Zoons E, Weisfelt M, de Gans J, Spanjaard L, Koelman JH, Reitsma JB, et al. Seizures in adults with bacterial meningitis. Neurology. 2008 May 27;70:2109–2115.
17. Vezzani A, Fujinami RS, White HS, Preux PM, Blumcke I, Sander JW, et al. Infections, inflammation and epilepsy. Acta Neuropathol. 2016 February;131:211–234.
18. Briand C, Levy C, Baumie F, Joao L, Bechet S, Carbonnelle E, et al. Outcomes of bacterial meningitis in children. Med. Mal. Infect. 2016 June;46:177–187.
19. Focke NK, Kallenberg K, Mohr A, Djukic M, Nau R, Schmidt H. Distributed, limbic gray matter atrophy in patients after bacterial meningitis. AJNR Am. J. Neuroradiol. 2013 June–July;34:1164–1167.
20. Bodilsen J, Dalager-Pedersen M, van de Beek D, Brouwer MC, Nielsen H. Long-term mortality and epilepsy in patients after brain abscess: a nationwide population-based matched cohort study. Clin. Infect. Dis. 2019 November 27;71:2825–2832.

21. Calliauw L, de Praetere P, Verbeke L. Postoperative epilepsy in subdural suppurations. Acta Neurochir (Wien). 1984;71:217–223.
22. Chuang MJ, Chang WN, Chang HW, Lin WC, Tsai NW, Hsieh MJ, et al. Predictors and long-term outcome of seizures after bacterial brain abscess. J. Neurol. Neurosurg. Psychiatry. 2010 August;81:913–917.
23. Bodilsen J, Duerlund LS, Mariager T, Brandt CT, Wiese L, Petersen PT, et al. Risk factors and prognosis of epilepsy following brain abscess: a nationwide population-based cohort study. Neurology. 2023 April 11;100:e1611–e1620.
24. Sinha S, Harish T, Taly AB, Murthy P, Nagarathna S, Chandramuki A. Symptomatic seizures in neurosyphilis: an experience from a university hospital in south India. Seizure. 2008 December;17:711–716.
25. Ramos AP, Burneo JG. Seizures and epilepsy associated with central nervous system tuberculosis. Seizure. 2023 April;107:60–66.
26. Misra UK, Kumar M, Kalita J. Seizures in tuberculous meningitis. Epilepsy Res. 2018 December;148:90–95.
27. Anjum N, Noureen N, Iqbal I. Clinical presentations and outcomes of the children with tuberculous meningitis: an experience at a tertiary care hospital. J. Pak. Med. Assoc. 2018 January;68:10–15.
28. Anderson NE, Somaratne J, Mason DF, Holland D, Thomas MG. Neurological and systemic complications of tuberculous meningitis and its treatment at Auckland City Hospital, New Zealand. J. Clin. Neurosci. 2010 September;17:1114–1118.
29. Segamwenge IL, Kioko NP, Mukulu C, Jacob O, Humphrey W, Augustinus J. Neurocysticercosis among patients with first time seizure in Northern Namibia. Pan Afr. Med. J. 2016;24:127.
30. Carpio A, Romo ML, Hauser WA, Kelvin EA. New understanding about the relationship among neurocysticercosis, seizures, and epilepsy. Seizure. 2021 August;90:123–129.
31. Satishchandra P, Sinha S. Seizures in HIV-seropositive individuals: NIMHANS experience and review. Epilepsia. 2008 August;49 Suppl 6:33–41.
32. Burman RJ, Wilmshurst JM, Gebauer S, Weise L, Walker KG, Donald KA. Seizures in children with HIV infection in South Africa: a retrospective case control study. Seizure. 2019 February;65:159–165.
33. Hung CW, Chang WN, Kung CT, Tsai NW, Wang HC, Lin WC, et al. Predictors and long-term outcome of seizures in human immuno-deficiency virus (HIV)-negative cryptococcal meningitis. BMC Neurol. 2014 October 13;14:208.
34. Alqwaifly M, Al-Ajlan FS, Al-Hindi H, Al Semari A. Central nervous system brucellosis granuloma and white matter disease in immunocompromised patient. Emerg. Infect. Dis. 2017 June;23:978–981.
35. Lucchese G. Herpesviruses, autoimmunity and epilepsy: peptide sharing and potential cross-reactivity with human synaptic proteins. Autoimmun. Rev. 2019 October;18:102367.
36. Wipfler P, Dunn N, Beiki O, Trinka E, Fogdell-Hahn A. The viral hypothesis of mesial temporal lobe epilepsy—is human herpes virus-6 the missing link? A systematic review and meta-analysis. Seizure. 2018 January;54:33–40.
37. Nash TE, Mahanty S, Loeb JA, Theodore WH, Friedman A, Sander JW, et al. Neurocysticercosis: a natural human model of epileptogenesis. Epilepsia. 2015 February; 56:177–183.
38. Walton D, Castell H, Collie C, Wood GK, Sharma M, Singh T, et al. Antiepileptic drugs for seizure control in people with neurocysticercosis. Cochrane Database Syst. Rev. 2021 November 1;11:CD009027.
39. Kirar RS, Uniyal R, Garg RK, Verma R, Malhotra HS, Sharma PK, et al. Occurrence and determinants of seizures and their impact on tuberculous meningitis: a prospective evaluation. Acta Neurol. Belg. 2024 June;124:821–829.

40. Kim MA, Park KM, Kim SE, Oh MK. Acute symptomatic seizures in CNS infection. Eur. J. Neurol. 2008 January;15:38–41.
41. Yang Q, Wei B. Risk factors of epilepsy secondary to viral encephalitis: a meta-analysis. J. Neuroimmunol. 2023 May 15;378:578089.
42. Hesdorffer DC, Benn EK, Cascino GD, Hauser WA. Is a first acute symptomatic seizure epilepsy? Mortality and risk for recurrent seizure. Epilepsia. 2009 May;50:1102–1108.
43. Singh AK, Garg RK, Rizvi I, Malhotra HS, Kumar N, Gupta RK. Clinical and neuroimaging predictors of seizure recurrence in solitary calcified neurocysticercosis: a prospective observational study. Epilepsy Res. 2017 November;137:78–83.
44. Elafros MA, Johnson BA, Siddiqi OK, Okulicz JF, Sikazwe I, Bositis CM, et al. Mortality & recurrent seizure risk after new-onset seizure in HIV-positive Zambian adults. BMC Neurol. 2018 December 7;18:201.
45. Olajumoke O, Akinsegun A, Njideka O, Oluwadamilola O, Olaitan O, Adedoyin D, et al. New- onset seizures in HIV patients on antiretroviral therapy at a tertiary centre in South-West, Nigeria. World J. Aids. 2013;3:67–70.
46. Chadha DS, Handa A, Sharma SK, Varadarajulu P, Singh AP. Seizures in patients with human immunodeficiency virus infection. J. Assoc. Physicians India. 2000 June;48:573–576.
47. Lachuriya G, Garg RK, Jain A, Malhotra HS, Singh AK, Jain B, et al. Toll-like receptor-4 polymorphisms and serum matrix metalloproteinase-9 in newly diagnosed patients with calcified neurocysticercosis and seizures. Medicine (Baltimore). 2016 April;95:e3288.
48. Sharma P, Garg RK, Verma R, Singh MK, Shukla R. Risk of seizure recurrence in patients of new-onset partial seizure having a solitary cysticercus granuloma of brain or normal neuroimaging. J. Neurol. Sci. 2011 February 15;301:21–26.
49. Rosman NP, Peterson DB, Kaye EM, Colton T. Seizures in bacterial meningitis: prevalence, patterns, pathogenesis, and prognosis. Pediatr. Neurol. 1985 September–October;1:278–285.
50. Pomeroy SL, Holmes SJ, Dodge PR, Feigin RD. Seizures and other neurologic sequelae of bacterial meningitis in children. N. Engl. J. Med. 1990 December 13;323:1651–1657.
51. Larsen F, Brandt CT, Larsen L, Klastrup V, Wiese L, Helweg-Larsen J, et al. Risk factors and prognosis of seizures in adults with community-acquired bacterial meningitis in Denmark: observational cohort studies. BMJ Open. 2019 July 1;9:e030263.
52. Hansen AE, Vestergaard HT, Dessau RB, Bodilsen J, Andersen NS, Omland LH, et al. Long-term survival, morbidity, social functioning and risk of disability in patients with a herpes simplex virus type 1 or type 2 central nervous system infection, Denmark, 2000–2016. Clin. Epidemiol. 2020;12:745–755.
53. Misra UK, Kalita J. Seizures in encephalitis: predictors and outcome. Seizure. 2009 October;18:583–587.
54. Lee S, Kim SH, Kim HD, Lee JS, Ko A, Kang HC. Identification of etiologies according to baseline clinical features of pediatric new-onset refractory status epilepticus in single center retrospective study. Seizure. 2024 June 12;120:49–55.
55. Leitinger M, Trinka E, Giovannini G, Zimmermann G, Florea C, Rohracher A, et al. Epidemiology of status epilepticus in adults: a population-based study on incidence, causes, and outcomes. Epilepsia. 2019 January;60:53–62.
56. Murthy JM, Prabhakar S. Bacterial meningitis and epilepsy. Epilepsia. 2008 August;49 Suppl 6:8–12.
57. Bianchi MT, Dworetzky BA, Bromfield EB. Auditory auras in patients with postencephalitic epilepsy: case series. Epilepsy Behav. 2009 January;14:250–252.
58. Singh G, Prabhakar S. The effects of antimicrobial and antiepileptic treatment on the outcome of epilepsy associated with central nervous system (CNS) infections. Epilepsia. 2008 August;49 Suppl 6:42–46.

59. Sharawat ID, Murugan VM, Bhardwaj SM, Tomar AD, Tiwari LM, Dhamija PD, et al. Efficacy and safety of phenytoin and levetiracetam for acute symptomatic seizures in children with acute encephalitis syndrome: an open label, randomised controlled trial. Seizure. 2024 May;118:110–116.

60. Birbeck GL, Herman ST, Capparelli EV, Dzinjalamala FK, Abdel Baki SG, Mallewa M, et al. A clinical trial of enteral Levetiracetam for acute seizures in pediatric cerebral malaria. BMC Pediatr. 2019 November 1;19:399.

61. Santhosh AP, Kumar Goyal M, Modi M, Kharbanda PS, Ahuja CK, Tandyala N, et al. Carbamazepine versus levetiracetam in epilepsy due to neurocysticercosis. Acta Neurol. Scand. 2021 March;143:242–247.

62. Sharawat IK, Panda PK, Kumar V, Sherwani P. Comparative efficacy and safety of lacosamide and oxcarbazepine for seizure control in children with newly diagnosed solitary neurocysticercosis. J. Trop. Pediatr. 2022 April 5;68:fmac032.

63. Beghi E, Giussani G, Grosso S, Iudice A, La Neve A, Pisani F, et al. Withdrawal of antiepileptic drugs: guidelines of the Italian League Against Epilepsy. Epilepsia. 2013 October;54 Suppl 7:2–12.

64. Sellner J, Trinka E. Clinical characteristics, risk factors and pre-surgical evaluation of post-infectious epilepsy. Eur. J. Neurol. 2013 March;20:429–439.

65. Fohlen M, Taussig D, Ferrand-Sorbets S, Maurey H, Petrescu A, Chipaux M, et al. Management and results of epilepsy surgery associated with acyclovir prophylaxis in four pediatric patients with drug-resistant epilepsy due to herpetic encephalitis and review of the literature. Eur. J. Paediatr. Neurol. 2020 November;29:128–136.

66. Liu S, Xiong Z, Wang J, Tang C, Deng J, Zhang J, et al. Efficacy and potential predictors of vagus nerve stimulation therapy in refractory postencephalitic epilepsy. Ther. Adv. Chronic Dis. 2022;13:20406223211066738.

67. Sun Y, Chen J, Fang T, Wan L, Shi X, Wang J, et al. Vagus nerve stimulation therapy for the treatment of seizures in refractory postencephalitic epilepsy: a retrospective study. Front. Neurosci. 2021;15:685685.

68. Pillai SC, Mohammad SS, Hacohen Y, Tantsis E, Prelog K, Barnes EH, et al. Postencephalitic epilepsy and drug-resistant epilepsy after infectious and antibody-associated encephalitis in childhood: clinical and etiologic risk factors. Epilepsia. 2016 January;57:e7–e11.

69. Xiong W, Lu L, Chen J, Xiao Y, Zhou D. Chronic post-encephalitic epilepsy following Japanese encephalitis: clinical features, neuroimaging data, and outcomes. Seizure. 2019 November;72:49–53.

70. de Almeida SM, Gurjao SA. Quality of life assessment in patients with neurocysticercosis. J. Community Health. 2011 August;36:624–630.

71. Zapata WR, Yang SY, Bustos JA, Gonzales I, Saavedra H, Guzman C, et al. Quality of life in patients with symptomatic epilepsy due to neurocysticercosis. Epilepsy Behav. 2022 June;131:108668.

72. Kvam KA, Stahl JP, Chow FC, Soldatos A, Tattevin P, Sejvar J, et al. Outcome and sequelae of infectious encephalitis. J. Clin. Neurol. 2024 January;20:23–36.

73. Forsgren L, Hauser WA, Olafsson E, Sander JW, Sillanpaa M, Tomson T. Mortality of epilepsy in developed countries: a review. Epilepsia. 2005;46 Suppl 11:18–27.

Immune-Mediated Epilepsy

5

5.1 RISK OF EPILEPSY

Immune-mediated epilepsy refers to epilepsy caused by an immunological reaction in the brain. The acute inflammation may cause acute symptomatic seizures, for instance during autoimmune encephalitis or a relapse of multiple sclerosis (MS). There is an ongoing debate if all seizures occurring during encephalitis are to be defined as acute symptomatic, as discussed later. Over time, immunological damage can result in epilepsy, a predisposition for seizures that remains also when the inflammation has subsided.

The last years have seen remarkable advances in the field of immune-mediated epilepsy, with more and more autoantibodies being detected as either pathogenic or indicators of disease. There is also an increased discussion regarding seronegative patients demonstrating a clinical presentation congruent with immune-mediated epilepsy; some of them could perhaps have encephalitis and benefit from immunotherapy.

5.1.1 Prevalence

It has been estimated that about 5% of all focal epilepsies of unknown cause may have an immunological cause.[1] Given that many cases probably go undetected, the actual figure may be higher. Autoimmune encephalitis seems more common than infectious encephalitis in many countries.[2] The prevalence of epilepsy in MS is around 2%, lower in aquaporin-associated disorders, but may be higher in myelin oligodendrocyte glycoprotein (MOG)-associated disease (Figure 5.1).[3] In reports of prevalence of all epilepsy, immune-mediated epilepsy is probably found in the other/undetermined category—accounting for less than 10% in total.[4]

5.1.2 Incidence

The incidence of immune-mediated epilepsy is difficult to determine. Case series from tertiary centers with an interest in the condition dominate the field, so publication

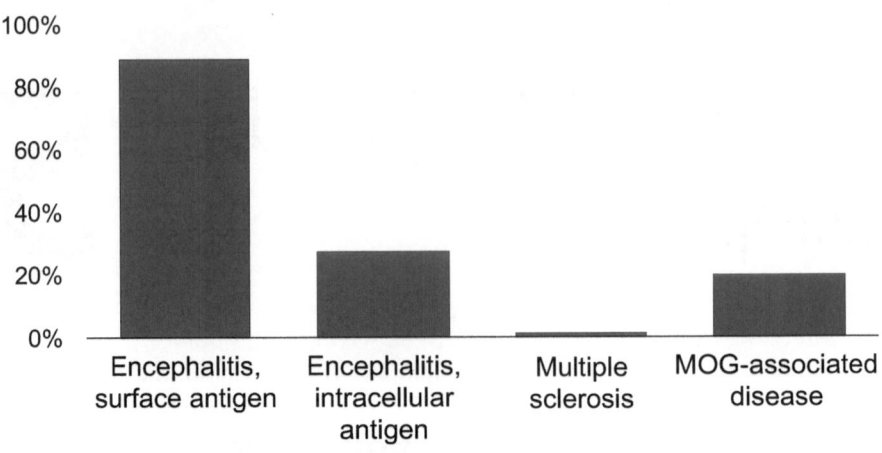

FIGURE 5.1   Prevalence of epilepsy in different immune disorders.

bias is likely. Seizures are often the presenting symptom in these studies, so patients with brain inflammation and no seizures are presumably treated elsewhere or remain undetected.

TERMINOLOGY

It has been suggested that the term autoimmune epilepsy should be reserved for cases with seizures occurring also after the initial inflammatory phase, in contrast to acute symptomatic seizures occurring while the autoimmune encephalitis is active.[2,5,6] This is indeed logical, but the terminology has not yet penetrated the clinic or all literature. Difficulties in applying the suggested terminology include the practical difficulties in determining when the inflammatory phase has ended. Biologically, the different phases in most cases of autoimmune encephalitis are presumably not mutually exclusive and immunological mechanisms may be involved in maintaining an ictogenic state beyond other encephalitis symtoms.[1] Inflammation or immune mechanisms may cause seizures in many different circumstances, from severe new-onset status epilepticus to cryptogenic focal epilepsy, and particularly in the latter case it may be difficult to determine if there is active inflammation going on or not. As a reader in the field, it is however good to be aware of the varying use of terminology—what some authors call epilepsy, others call acute symptomatic seizures.

5.1.3 Risk in Different Conditions

The risk of immune-mediated epilepsy varies with the inflammatory condition. Idiopathic and paraneoplastic autoimmune encephalitis are the most well-known immune etiologies, but multiple sclerosis can also fulfill the definition of an immunological cause. Additionally, all autoimmune systemic disorders increase the risk of epilepsy—suggesting that a person's immunological responses may facilitate epileptogenic processes and illustrating how little we still understand of this complex matter. To further complicate matters, systemic inflammation in general (for instance in cases of infection) can aggravate preexisting epilepsy. That inflammation can also facilitate ictogenesis of course makes studies of the involvement in epileptogenesis very complicated.

5.1.4 Autoimmune Encephalitis

Autoimmune encephalitis is traditionally divided into paraneoplastic and non-paraneoplastic cases, and into encephalitis with antibodies against neuronal surface and intracellular antigens. In both groups the risk of seizures during the acute encephalitis phase varies with the antigen; some antibodies carry a particularly high seizure risk. Some clinical characteristics are presented in Table 5.1.

Autoantibodies against surface antigens (for instance NMDA receptors, GABA receptors, etc.) have a higher risk of seizures in the acute stage, in some case series up to 100%, but these could have a lower risk of later epilepsy because they tend to cause neuronal dysfunction rather than brain damage (see Epileptogenesis section).[1] These antibodies cause seizures and other symptoms if administered intrathecally in animal experiments and affect neuronal function *in vitro*. There may be triggers like previous viral encephalitis. In NMDA-receptor or LGI1-receptor encephalitis, a very high proportion have seizures during the acute phase.[2]

Cases of autoimmune encephalitis by antibodies directed against intracellular antigens, including the often paraneoplastic onconeural antibodies, can also have seizures as a symptom of acute encephalitis. These encephalitides seem more prone to cause structural damage and later epilepsy. In many cases—it is not certain that the antibodies themselves are the cause of the brain damage—they may be markers of tissue destruction.

TABLE 5.1   Antibodies Often Associated with Seizures

ANTIBODY (ANTI-)	CLINICAL FEATURES
NMDA	Psychiatric symptoms, movement disorder, autonomic dysfunction. Ovarian teratoma in women.
GABA$_A$	Status epilepticus.
GABA$_B$	Limbic encephalitis, seizures.
LGI1	Limbic encephalitis, faciobrachial dystonic seizures. Hyponatremia.
Caspr2	Peripheral nerve symptoms, limbic encephalitis, ataxia.

5.1.5 Multiple Sclerosis and Similar Disorders

Multiple sclerosis is an autoimmune inflammatory disorder that most often does not cause acute seizures during the inflammation of relapses, although exceptions exist. In most cases, MS seems to cause epilepsy by accumulating damage to brain networks. Approximately 3% of MS patients develop epilepsy. Seizures typically arise later in the disease course and in the progressive phase,[7–9] suggesting that structural damage underlies this particular immune-mediated epilepsy. The low risk of epilepsy in MS has clinical importance, since it may prevent erroneous epilepsy diagnoses in patients with early/mild MS who have had only one seizure (see Risk of Epilepsy after a First Unprovoked Seizure section). Some reviews suggest a difference in geographic prevalence of epilepsy in MS, with particularly investigations from Asia reporting higher rates.[3]

Other neuroinflammatory diseases like MOG-associated disorders and aquaporin-associated disorders have been less extensively studied than MS. The prevalence seems lower in aquaporin-associated disorders like neuromyolitis optica, but up to 20% have been reported to have epilepsy in MOG-associated disorders.[3]

5.1.6 Autoimmune Epilepsy and Epilepsy in Systemic Inflammation

The increased awareness of autoimmune encephalitis causing epilepsy has given rise to discussions about pure autoimmune epilepsy, a concept referring to epilepsy caused by inflammation without other associated features of limbic encephalitis. Antibodies against brain tissue are detected in up to 10% of new-onset epilepsy cases,[10–14] and there are case reports of temporal lobe epilepsy as the first paraneoplastic symptom, which offers theoretical support to the concept of autoimmune epilepsy. More information is needed. A distinction between very mild autoimmune encephalitis and pure autoimmune epilepsy is perhaps theoretical.

Epilepsy can arise in any inflammatory condition, like in Hashimoto thyroiditis, in vasculitis, and after infections, but the involvement of immune mechanisms is often not clear.[15,16]

5.2 EPILEPTOGENESIS

The neurobiology underlying seizures in immune-mediated epilepsy is fascinating, and the knowledge on epileptogenesis evolves rapidly. Briefly, antibodies against neuronal antigens can cause tissue inflammation involving both T-cells and the innate immune system, but tissue damage can also lead to exposure of neuronal antigens and autoantibodies that are disease markers rather than pathogenic. The inflammation can also cause structural damage, which disrupts networks and leads to epilepsy.[1]

HISTORY OF AUTOIMMUNE ENCEPHALITIS

Autoimmune encephalitis was described in the 1960s as paraneoplastic limbic encephalitis. The triad of cognitive impairment, psychiatric symptoms, and seizures were identified hallmark features, and the subacute onset with a high seizure frequency was also noted.[17] The discovery of antibodies associated with paraneoplastic limbic encephalitis allowed a link between the immune and nervous system (these included Hu, Ma2/Ta, amphiphysin, VGCC, and mGluR5, which were later found not to be pathogenic, but biomarkers). About 20 years ago, non-paraneoplastic cases emerged in the literature,[18] and non-paraneoplastic cases are now believed to be the more common form.

5.2.1 The Role of Antibodies

In NMDAR-autoimmune encephalitis, antibodies bind to the NMDA receptor and as a result reduce the excitation of inhibitory neurons in the basal ganglia and limbic system, which causes seizures, psychiatric symptoms, and more. Similarly, anti-LGI1- and AMPA-receptor antibodies are believed to cause hyperexcitability of neuronal circuits by binding to their targets and changing neuronal function. Anti-LGI1 antibodies seem to have effect both at the initial axon segment, where action potentials are generated, and presynaptically in glutamatergic synapses. Some antibodies, like GABA-A-receptor antibodies, are believed to reduce inhibitory inputs by antagonistically blocking postsynaptic receptors. GAD antibodies on the other hand are thought to interfere with the conversion of glutamate to GABA. This could theoretically cause reduced GABA and an excess of glutamate in many synapses, but since GAD is an intracellular enzyme, the exact mechanisms are not understood.[1] GAD antibodies are associated with many other symptoms, like stiff person syndrome, but what underlies the variable presentations in different cases also remains elusive.

It is not clear if antibodies need to be produced intrathecally to cause or indicate autoimmune encephalitis. Theoretically, antibody-producing B-cells could reside in the periphery and the antibodies cross into the brain with blood–brain barrier disruption, or B-cells could cross into the CNS resulting in intrathecal production. Some patients with clinical autoimmune encephalitis are antibody positive in blood, others in CSF, and many in both. In double-positive patients, the titers are usually higher in blood. To complicate matters further, the brain has been suggested to function as an immunoprecipitant—meaning that antibodies may bind to tissue but not be that detectable in fluids.[2] An interesting speculation is if the locality of production could be one explanation for why only some patients respond to plasma exchange.[1]

Finally, it seems that certain antibody-mediated encephalitis (LGI1 and CASPR2) almost only occurs in patients with certain HLA types.[2] This has been suggested to perhaps reflect vulnerability in the B-T-cell interaction needed for antibody production.

5.2.2 The Role of the Innate Immune System

The innate immune system involves complement and microglia activation, among other processes. In the brain, the innate system can cause tissue damage but also induce changes in neurons. For instance, many studies have demonstrated increased levels of IL-1ß after seizures, which alters neuronal expression of receptors and leads to hyperexcitability. Other possible mechanisms could be immune complexes causing vascular changes.[1] There is also preclinical evidence emerging that cytokine profiles may influence neurons or glia to more pro- or anti-ictogenic states. An interesting concept is genetic vulnerability through inflammatory mechanisms; genetic variability in IL-1ß SNPs has been associated with both autoimmune disorders and temporal lobe epilepsy.[19] Similarly, epidemiological data suggest a clear overrepresentation of epilepsy among patients with non-neurological autoimmune diseases.[20]

5.2.3 Time Course

It can be helpful to make a distinction between the encephalitis phase with active brain inflammation and later phases with only epilepsy. Onset is typically rapid, with symptoms reaching the maximum in days or weeks.[2,21] Sometimes, it may even be new-onset refractory status epilepticus (NORSE), in which status epilepticus is the presenting symptom at the onset of encephalitis in a previously healthy individual. Some patients with immune-medicated epilepsy may have a high seizure frequency for months, but then enter remission. The high initial seizure frequency, as well as the remission, is rare in epilepsy caused by most structural lesions discussed in the rest of the book and supports the notion that active inflammation may either cause or perpetuate seizures. The length of the initial inflammatory period probably varies, but immunotherapy seems most effective soon after onset, which may give some indication to the time scale involved. Clinical scores trying to predict response to immunotherapy also incorporate elapsed time from symptom onset to therapy start (less is better), suggesting that inflammation needs to be treated rapidly.

5.2.4 White Matter Demyelination in MS and Similar Disorders

In MS and related disorders like neuromyelitis optica (NMO) or MOG-associated inflammation, theories of epileptogenesis include disruption of networks rather than direct effects on neurons. However, demyelination is believed to cause ion displacement, metabolic stress, and mitochondrial dysfunction, which may cause hyperexcitability as well as start neurodegeneration.[3]

5.2.5 Inflammation as a Perpetuating Mechanism in Other Epilepsies?

Immune mechanisms are probably also involved in seizures and epilepsy outside of the traditional autoimmune encephalitides. For instance, numerous studies have found increased levels of inflammatory markers in blood or CSF in patients with high seizure frequency. This is particularly the case for IL6, Toll-like receptor 4, and HMGBox 1 signaling—which are all involved in the innate immune system. Status epilepticus or medically refractory epilepsy can at least seem steroid responsive,[22] which should perhaps not be interpreted as evidence that inflammation causes seizures but raises a possibility that an inflammatory state can facilitate them. Which patient groups merit trials of immunotherapy is not known, nor is the best modality of treatment.

5.3 RISK FACTORS

Because inflammation is a less recognizable entity than traumatic brain injury or stroke, there are very few cohort studies allowing a proper understanding of risk factors. What is becoming known and most helpful for a clinician are risk factors for an immune-mediated cause in patients with epilepsy. The presentation is variable, but risk factors that should raise suspicion are subacute onset of seizures, high seizure frequency, memory decline, altered level of consciousness, psychiatric symptoms, autonomic dysregulation, or specific seizure types like faciobrachial dystonic seizures in LGI1 autoimmune encephalitis (Table 5.2).

In MS, evidence suggests that epilepsy often arises because of the structural damage caused by the inflammation. The risk of epilepsy is closely correlated to the accumulated disability and duration of disease. For individuals in the national Swedish MS register, epilepsy was more common in cases of secondary progressive MS than in the earlier phase of relapsing remitting MS. The risk increased with age, disability score, and MS duration.[8,23]

TABLE 5.2   Risk Factors That Should Raise Suspicion of Immune-Mediated Epilepsy

- Subacute onset
- High seizure frequency
- Memory decline or altered level of consciousness
- Psychiatric symptoms
- Autonomic dysregulation
- Specific seizure types

5.3.1 Risk of Epilepsy after Acute Symptomatic Seizures

Acute symptomatic seizures occur in several autoimmune encephalitides, like NMDA-receptor and CASPR2 autoimmune encephalitis. In some cases, the acute symptomatic seizure may be severe as in NORSE. The risk of chronic epilepsy varies and seems lower after LG1-associated encephalitis than that after GAD65-associated encephalitis. A relatively high risk (at least 30%) of chronic epilepsy is described for cases of NORSE.[24]

5.3.2 Risk of Epilepsy after a First Unprovoked Seizure

5.3.2.1 Autoimmune Encephalitis

In autoimmune encephalitis detected after the first tonic-clonic seizure, the risk of seizure recurrence is extremely high. In clinical practice, recurrence risk is rarely an issue since there is usually a high frequency of focal seizures that have preceded or followed the tonic-clonic seizure.[21] Careful history taking about subtle signs is however important; it is not uncommon for patients to ignore feelings of epigastric rising, déjà vu, or piloerection until prompted. In clear cases of autoimmune encephalitis, focal seizures can occur several times per day. The important aspect is not just that early detection allows rapid instigation of ASM treatment, but that it may allow immunotherapy. Clinicians should therefore be on the lookout for signs that could suggest an autoimmune origin in new-onset seizure patients (Table 5.2).

5.3.2.2 Multiple Sclerosis and Related Disorders

Onset of epilepsy in MS is most often in the form of unprovoked seizures, occurring without relation to an acute relapse. Some exceptions have been reported, in which seizures were at least temporally associated with MS relapses and subsided with disease-modifying therapy.[25] Judging from Swedish register data, the recurrence risk after a first unprovoked seizure in MS varies with disease state (Figure 5.2). In relapsing remitting MS, the risk of seizure recurrence is not different from that of random controls (around 40% at 10 years), whereas patients experiencing a first seizure in secondary progressive MS have a 61% (95% CI 47%–75%) risk of epilepsy. The risk seems particularly high after status epilepticus: 82% (95% CI 68%–100%).[26] There are methodological caveats with register studies, mainly difficulties in determining accuracy of diagnoses, but the risk of seizure recurrence certainly seems high after status epilepticus in MS. There is insufficient data about aquaporin- and MOG-associated disorders concerning recurrence risks after a first seizure.

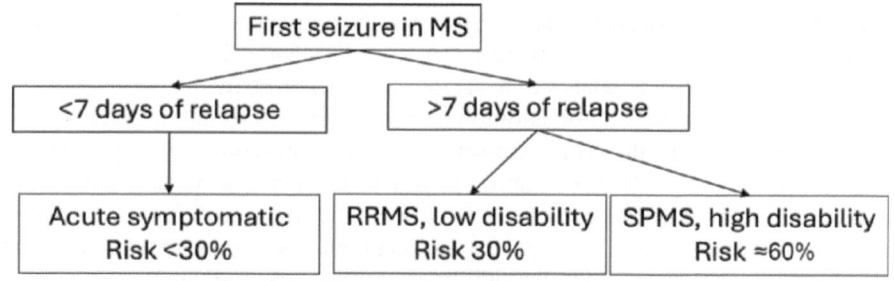

FIGURE 5.2   Recurrence risk after a first seizure in multiple sclerosis.

5.3.2.3 Other Inflammatory Diseases

Although several studies have demonstrated an increased risk of epilepsy in patients with systemic inflammatory diseases or other autoimmune conditions, there is currently no data to suggest that a first unprovoked seizure in such circumstances merits any specific management or entails a particularly high risk of recurrence. If there are brain lesions, which is rare, the risk is higher.

5.4 MANAGEMENT

5.4.1 Clinical Presentation

5.4.1.1 Autoimmune Encephalitis

In classic autoimmune encephalitis, the onset of epilepsy is often close to the onset of the inflammation. Presentation is rapid, over days to weeks, but exceptions extending into years exist.[2] Current expert opinion suggests that suspicion of mild limbic encephalitis should be raised when seizure frequency is high, together with cognitive impairment and psychiatric symptoms.[27,28] The response to antiseizure medication is typically suboptimal, and many patients demonstrate refractoriness unless immunotherapy is started.[29] The psychiatric symptoms can be very diverse, from mood disorders to psychotic symptoms of varying degrees.[2] The typical example is NMDA-receptor encephalitis, in which psychiatric symptoms can dominate in milder cases and seizures only emerge later, if at all. Cognitive symptoms may range from confusion to amnesia.

The seizures can sometimes point to the autoantibody involved. Faciobrachial dystonic seizures are typical of LGI1-antibody encephalitis, but the patients often have multiple focal seizure types, including piloerection seizures. Tonic-clonic seizures may ensue.[2] Focal seizures are also common in CASPR2-antibody encephalitis. Status epilepticus is frequent in patients with GABA-receptor antibodies. Many autoimmune encephalitides show movement disorders in addition to seizures. Dyskinesias of the mouth, rigidity, dystonia, and gait disturbance as well as ataxia have been described, as have autonomic symptoms related to heart rate or blood pressure.[2]

Overall, the heterogeneity of autoimmune conditions is substantial, and cases range from those identified in the outpatient setting to those presenting as refractory status epilepticus. New-onset refractory status epilepticus is a heterogeneous condition, with refractory SE without any detectable etiology being the common denominator. There is sometimes a preceding febrile illness. In status epilepticus in general it is important to pursue etiology and consider the possibility of encephalitis, and whether this is infectious or autoimmune. CSF analysis is needed.[30] Differential diagnoses to an autoimmune cause often include glioma, infectious encephalitis, Creutzfeldt–Jakob disease (CJD), or metabolic conditions, and most diagnostic algorithms for NORSE describe ways to exclude these. In NMDA-receptor encephalitis, EEG may show extreme delta brush and there may be mild CSF lymphocytosis.

5.4.1.2 Multiple Sclerosis and Similar Disorders

Presentation is usually at a relatively advanced disease stage. Sometimes there are difficulties differentiating focal seizures from spasticity or other subcortical paroxysmal symptoms. It may be prudent to exclude an MS relapse as a cause of a first seizure in a person with MS—this is rare but may indicate a need for more aggressive MS therapy.

CASE 5.1 First Seizure in MS

A 35-year-old man has a first tonic-clonic seizure. Two years ago, he was diagnosed with multiple sclerosis after an episode of opticus neuritis, his MRI showed two lesions, and CSF showed oligoclonal bands. He is on oral disease modifying therapy. Because of the seizure he undergoes a rapid MRI with MS protocol, but there is no evidence of a relapse. At the first seizure clinic, he inquires about recurrence risk.

Comment: A first seizure in relapsing remitting MS is not definitely associated with an increased risk of epilepsy compared to controls. The counselling of this patient should be like for any other first unprovoked seizure—meaning that in five years the risk of epilepsy (seizure recurrence) is about 40–50%.

5.4.1.3 Suspecting Inflammation in Epilepsy of Unknown Cause

Other than staying vigilant for associated symptoms suggesting autoimmune encephalitis, there is yet no certain evidence suggesting that clinicians should suspect all cryptogenic epilepsy of having an immunological etiology. Screening for antibodies in all cases of new-onset seizures is not possible, nor perhaps advisable.[2] The situation changes if there are other symptoms (Table 5.3). In cases of intractable focal epilepsy

TABLE 5.3   Factors That Have Been Identified as Predictors of Positive Antibody Testing[31,32]

New-onset status epilepticus or seizure cluster
Progressive altered mental status
Autonomic dysfunction
Viral prodrome
Particular seizure types (facial dyskinesias/faciobrachial dystonic)
Focal CNS findings
Autoimmune disorder
MRI changes
Malignancy
Systemic factors (weight loss, hyponatremia, peripheral nerve hyperexcitability)

and associated neurocognitive symptoms, the likelihood of finding neuronal antibodies seems quite high—around 10%–20% at tertiary centers.[33,34] A clinical antibody prevalence in epilepsy score has been developed that aims to assist identification of patients that may benefit from antibody testing.[34] Age >54, ictal piloerection, self-reported lower mood, MRI changes in the limbic system, absence of epilepsy risk factors, and intact attention predicted presence of antibodies according to another study.[14]

5.4.2 Treatment

Treatment for immune epilepsy is currently based on expert opinion and rests on clinical experience as well as some initial studies, most of which are observational.

5.4.2.1 Screening for Malignancy

If an autoimmune encephalitis is suspected, some sort of malignancy screening is generally advised. In larger series at least 20% of women with NMDA-receptor antibodies and autoimmune encephalitis have an ovarian teratoma, and paraneoplastic status epilepticus has been described in a wide range of tumors.[21] In addition to whole-body imaging and careful systems review, different antibodies can point to different malignancies, like small cell lung cancer or breast cancer, indicating systems in need of closer imaging or other investigations.

5.4.2.2 Immunotherapy in the Acute Phase of Acute Encephalitis

The most important disease-modifying treatment in non-paraneoplastic autoimmune epilepsy is probably immunotherapy, which is reliant on recognition of the clinical syndrome. The first-line treatment at least in European centers is often corticosteroids,[35] followed by IVIG or plasma exchange, but some authorities suggest early combinations in more severe cases.[2] These initial steps are sometimes followed by anti-CD20 treatment or other immunotherapies. The field is rapidly advancing and cases should be managed at expert centers. It is probably important not to delay initial immunotherapy, at least corticosteroids, IVIG or plasma exchange is often tried relatively rapidly if the suspicion of an immune cause is high and initial immunotherapy considered safe.[2]

There are many interesting immune therapies emerging. Among these are several that target B-cells and T-cells selectively or elements of the inflammatory response like interleukin-6, interleukin-1, and TNF-alpha.[36] Selection of the optimal therapy beyond first-line treatment with steroids, IvIG, or plasma exchange is best done at tertiary centers. There are clinical scores that can be used to predict the response to immunotherapy.[1]

5.4.2.3 Immunotherapy in Medially Refractory Epilepsy

In careful assessment of medically refractory epilepsy, some have a history suggestive of previous autoimmune encephalitis. There is only expert opinion on how long encephalitis may still be present after the onset of seizures, and therefore how long the epilepsy may be responsive to immunotherapy. New-onset seizures and a shorter latency from symptom onset to immunotherapy is integral to scores predicting immunotherapy response,[32] so one might speculate that there is a more active period with regards to inflammation in the first year or so, in which immunotherapy is more effective. Clinical trials have examined the response to corticosteroids or IVIG in some cases of medically refractory epilepsy (Table 5.4). Most of these studies were uncontrolled and therefore vulnerable to various bias, but taken together they indicate a need for more research. Expert opinion seems to be that immunotherapy works best in patients with other, albeit sometimes mild, features of autoimmune encephalitis in addition to seizures.[37]

TABLE 5.4   Immune Therapy of Diagnosed or Suspected Immune-Mediated Epilepsy

IMMUNOTHERAPY OF EPILEPSY, SELECTED STUDIES	
RANDOMIZED TRIALS	
STUDY	*RESULT*
Dubey et al. 2020[38]	IvIg reduced seizures in LGI1/CASPR2 epilepsy more than placebo.
OBSERVATIONAL STUDIES	
STUDY	*RESULT*
Falsaperla et al. 2024[22]	Corticosteroids for three days had 63% responder rate in children with drug-resistant epilepsy.
Kimizu et al. 2020[39]	Methylprednisolone pulse therapy gave 32% responder rate in drug-resistant epilepsy.
von Rhein 2017[40]	46% responders in patients with suspected antibody-negative autoimmune limbic encephalitis.
Toledano et al. 2014[41]	Corticosteroids and/or IVIG in presumed autoimmune epilepsy resulted in 62% responders.

5.4.2.4 Combining ASMs with Immunotherapy

Immunotherapy is associated in time with seizure freedom or markedly improved seizure frequency.[21,29] The response rates vary between case series, but immunotherapy is often needed to stop seizures in addition to ASMs. In LGI1 encephalitis, some authors report faciobrachial seizures stopping only in 10% with ASMs in contrast to much better response to immunotherapy.[2] In some cases, focal seizures may be acceptable while immunotherapy response is awaited to avoid excessive ASM drug load, and some authors report a high incidence of cutaneous side effects in patients with LGI1 encephalitis,[42] so extensive polytherapy may carry additional risk in this particular epilepsy. The response to immunotherapy is often prompt, but may take months.[2,21]

5.4.2.5 Selecting ASM

There is no high-grade evidence regarding choice of ASM in autoimmune encephalitis. Observational studies suggest that sodium channel blockers may be most effective, but frequent combination therapy and the observational nature of these reports prevent definite conclusions (Table 5.5).[29,42,43]

Seizures in the acute phase are treated in the same manner as other acute symptomatic seizures. In the outpatient setting the ASMs most suitable are those that rapidly titrated to an effective dose: examples include levetiracetam, valproic acid, and lacosamide. Strong CYP450 inducers like phenytoin and carbamazepine are probably best avoided since they may interfere with the immunotherapy.[1] A survey of European centers showed that levetiracetam was the most common first-line ASM in immune epilepsy, and that lamotrigine, lacosamide, valproate, and carbamazepine were common second-line choices.[35]

5.4.2.6 ASM Withdrawal

Not all patients with seizures caused by autoimmune encephalitis have epilepsy once the inflammation has been treated or subsided.[2] Predicting who will tolerate ASM

TABLE 5.5 Antiseizure Medications in Immune-Mediated Epilepsy

ANTISEIZURE MEDICATION IN IMMUNE-MEDIATED EPILEPSY, SELECTED STUDIES	
OBSERVATIONAL STUDIES	
STUDY	RESULT
Feyissa et al. 2017[43]	Sodium-channel blockers (carbamazepine, oxcarbazepine, lacosamide, phenytoin) were used in a few patients who became seizure free, which was not the case for levetiracetam. Most also received immunotherapy.
Uribe-San-Martin et al. 2020[42]	Carbamazepine preceded seizure reduction in six patients with LGI1-antibody associated epilepsy. Most also received immunotherapy.

withdrawal is difficult in general and in narrow epilepsy populations in particular. Unfortunately, there is currently no robust evidence identifying individual patients with particularly low risk of seizure recurrence, but one study found that patients with previous autoimmune encephalitis and antibodies against surface antigens (NMDA, LGI1, Caspr2) had a much higher likelihood of final remission than patients with antibodies against intracellular antigens (GAD, Ma2),[44] suggesting that the former is the group in which ASM withdrawal could be attempted if the patient so desires after information about the risks of seizure recurrence.

As discussed in the introduction, patients with immune-mediated epilepsy are in need of better data for accurate prognostication. Systematically collected data are needed to avoid misdiagnosis of epilepsy when seizures have in fact been acute symptomatic due to an inflammation that has been cured. This becomes even more important, since the literature suggests that more patients with an insidious disease course or antibody negativity are likely to be identified and treated in the future. In the future, more precise knowledge on the immunological processes as well as assessment of tissue damage may allow better predictive models.[45]

5.4.2.7 Status Epilepticus

In status epilepticus, management follows the general staged approach. Autoimmune encephalitis is believed to underlie a relatively large proportion of new-onset refractory status epilepticus, and a consensus statement advocates rapid instigation of inflammatory treatment.[46] In status epilepticus, most European centers in a survey preferred levetiracetam and valproate before phenytoin as their ASM after benzodiazepines,[35] but in severe cases combination therapy is usually attempted just like in other etiologies. The important part is rapid instigation of immunotherapy as soon as infectious causes have been reasonably excluded, in addition to the treatment of seizures.

5.4.2.8 Epilepsy in Multiple Sclerosis

There are no randomized controlled trials comparing different ASMs in multiple sclerosis. In a study on Swedish prescription register data, we found lamotrigine as a first ASM to have slightly lower risk of discontinuation than carbamazepine, which is in agreement with the literature on focal epilepsy in general.[50] Other observational data suggest that there are no major differences in effectiveness between ASMs.[23] In rare cases of relapsing remitting MS, seizure frequency has been reported to be related to inflammatory activity and responsive to more aggressive MS treatment.[25] In such cases, there are hopefully other markers of MS activity as well.

5.4.2.9 Other Symptoms

Associated symptoms in autoimmune encephalitis is best treated in cooperation with psychiatric consults. Neuroleptic drugs as well as benzodiazepines can be beneficial for psychiatric symptoms and movement disorders, but therapy needs to be individualized.[2]

5.4.3 Non-Medical Treatment

Ketogenic diet is part of the protocol for severe cases of pediatric NORSE and may act partly through immunomodulation.[1,46] In epilepsy surgery work-up, autoantibodies may suggest that an immune-mediated etiology has been missed, and in some cases immunotherapy could be attempted before surgery.[1] The evidence is scarce, so management must be on a case-by-case basis.

5.5 PROGNOSIS

5.5.1 Seizures

5.5.1.1 Autoimmune Encephalitis

Important prognostic issues in the management of seizures in autoimmune epilepsy is the risk of continued seizures and the proportion developing pharmacoresistant epilepsy (Table 5.6). This seems to vary with the cause of epilepsy. Autoimmune encephalitis with antibodies against surface antigens carries the best epilepsy prognosis, whereas those with antibodies against intracellular antigens seem to do worse.[1,2] The matter is further complicated by the fact that the encephalitis may also relapse and with it seizures, a phenomenon reported in about a third of cases at large centers,[1] but the proportion probably varies with the case mix. If seizures do continue, drug resistance does not seem more common than in epilepsy in general. In one series, only 16% developed drug-resistant epilepsy.[47] Risk factors were status epilepticus (odds ratio 2), temporal lobe semiology (OR 10), and periodic discharges on the admission EEG (OR 20).

TABLE 5.6 Clinical Take-Home Messages

- Immune-mediated epilepsy is increasingly recognized. Autoimmune encephalitis is an important cause, and pathogenic antibodies are not always identified.
- Inflammatory brain diseases like MS may also cause epilepsy, and the risk increases like for all structural epilepsies. A first seizure in mild MS may not indicate a higher recurrence risk than after any first seizure.
- Recognition of the clinical phenotype is important; indicators may be high seizure frequency at onset, psychiatric symptoms or altered mental status, particular seizure types, MRI changes, and systemic signs like hyponatremia.
- Immunotherapy is important, perhaps more important than antiseizure medications in achieving remission. Steroids, Ivig, and more advanced therapies are used and selected on an individual basis.

5.5.1.2 Multiple Sclerosis and Other Neuroinflammatory Conditions

In MS, observational studies suggest that at least half of patients become seizure free with ASM in mono- or combination therapy.[23] This is slightly lower than expected for epilepsy in general, in which only one third become pharmacoresistant. Whether this is because of actual pharmacoresistance or low ambitions in epilepsy care is not known. Epilepsy in patients with MS is associated with increased mortality. An important confounder is probably the disease severity, but contribution of seizure-related risks and ASM side effects are hard to rule out.[48]

Epilepsy in NMO-spectrum and similar disorders have been much less studied.

5.5.2 Cognition

Because autoimmune epilepsy is a relatively new concept, data on cognitive outcomes are only just beginning to emerge. Some reviews recommend repeated cognitive assessment as a means of monitoring for disease recurrence.[49]

REFERENCES

1. Flammer J, Neziraj T, Ruegg S, Probstel AK. Immune mechanisms in epileptogenesis: update on diagnosis and treatment of autoimmune epilepsy syndromes. Drugs. 2023 February;83:135–158.
2. Uy CE, Binks S, Irani SR. Autoimmune encephalitis: clinical spectrum and management. Pract. Neurol. 2021 October;21:412–423.
3. Li EC, Zheng Y, Cai MT, Lai QL, Fang GL, Du BQ, et al. Seizures and epilepsy in multiple sclerosis, aquaporin 4 antibody-positive neuromyelitis optica spectrum disorder, and myelin oligodendrocyte glycoprotein antibody-associated disease. Epilepsia. 2022 September;63:2173–2191.
4. Syvertsen M, Nakken KO, Edland A, Hansen G, Hellum MK, Koht J. Prevalence and etiology of epilepsy in a Norwegian county: a population based study. Epilepsia. 2015 May;56:699–706.
5. Steriade C, Britton J, Dale RC, Gadoth A, Irani SR, Linnoila J, et al. Acute symptomatic seizures secondary to autoimmune encephalitis and autoimmune-associated epilepsy: conceptual definitions. Epilepsia. 2020 July;61:1341–1351.
6. Rada A, Bien CG. What is autoimmune encephalitis-associated epilepsy? Proposal of a practical definition. Epilepsia. 2023 June 23;64:2249–2255.
7. Martinez-Juarez IE, Lopez-Meza E, Gonzalez-Aragon Mdel C, Ramirez-Bermudez J, Corona T. Epilepsy and multiple sclerosis: increased risk among progressive forms. Epilepsy Res. 2009 April;84:250–253.
8. Burman J, Zelano J. Epilepsy in multiple sclerosis: a nationwide population-based register study. Neurology. 2017 December 12;89:2462–2468.
9. Gasparini S, Ferlazzo E, Ascoli M, Sueri C, Cianci V, Russo C, et al. Risk factors for unprovoked epileptic seizures in multiple sclerosis: a systematic review and meta-analysis. Neurol. Sci. 2017 March;38:399–406.

10. Zelano J, Axelsson M, Constantinescu R, Malmestrom C, Kumlien E. Neuronal antibodies in adult patients with new-onset seizures: a prospective study. Brain Behav. 2019 November;9:e01442.
11. Garcia-Tarodo S, Datta AN, Ramelli GP, Marechal-Rouiller F, Bien CG, Korff CM. Circulating neural antibodies in unselected children with new-onset seizures. Eur. J. Paediatr. Neurol. 2018 May;22:396–403.
12. Elisak M, Krysl D, Hanzalova J, Volna K, Bien CG, Leypoldt F, et al. The prevalence of neural antibodies in temporal lobe epilepsy and the clinical characteristics of seropositive patients. Seizure. 2018 December;63:1–6.
13. Suleiman J, Wright S, Gill D, Brilot F, Waters P, Peacock K, et al. Autoantibodies to neuronal antigens in children with new-onset seizures classified according to the revised ILAE organization of seizures and epilepsies. Epilepsia. 2013 December;54:2091–2100.
14. McGinty RN, Handel A, Moloney T, Ramesh A, Fower A, Torzillo E, et al. Clinical features which predict neuronal surface autoantibodies in new-onset focal epilepsy: implications for immunotherapies. J. Neurol. Neurosurg. Psychiatry. 2021 March;92:291–294.
15. Varrasi C, Vecchio D, Magistrelli L, Strigaro G, Tassi L, Cantello R. Auditory seizures in autoimmune epilepsy: a case with anti-thyroid antibodies. Epileptic. Disord. 2017 March 1;19:99–103.
16. Makhija P, Gopinath S, Kannoth S, Radhakrishnan K. A case of post-leptospirosis autoimmune epilepsy presenting with sleep-related hypermotor seizures. Epileptic. Disord. 2017 November 21;19:456–460.
17. Gaspard N. Autoimmune epilepsy. Continuum (Minneap. Minn.). 2016 February;22:227–245.
18. Vincent A, Buckley C, Schott JM, Baker I, Dewar BK, Detert N, et al. Potassium channel antibody-associated encephalopathy: a potentially immunotherapy-responsive form of limbic encephalitis. Brain. 2004 March;127:701–712.
19. Malekpour M, Salarikia SR, Kashkooli M, Asadi-Pooya AA. The genetic link between systemic autoimmune disorders and temporal lobe epilepsy: a bioinformatics study. Epilepsia Open. 2023 June;8:509–516.
20. Ong MS, Kohane IS, Cai T, Gorman MP, Mandl KD. Population-level evidence for an autoimmune etiology of epilepsy JAMA Neurol. 2014 May;71: 569 –574.
21. de Bruijn M, van Sonderen A, van Coevorden-Hameete MH, Bastiaansen AEM, Schreurs MWJ, Rouhl RPW, et al. Evaluation of seizure treatment in anti-LGI1, anti-NMDAR, and anti-GABA(B)R encephalitis. Neurology. 2019 May 7;92:e2185–e2196.
22. Falsaperla R, Collotta AD, Marino SD, Sortino V, Leonardi R, Privitera GF, et al. Drug resistant epilepsies: a multicentre case series of steroid therapy. Seizure. 2024 February 13;117:115–125.
23. Dagiasi I, Vall V, Kumlien E, Burman J, Zelano J. Treatment of epilepsy in multiple sclerosis. Seizure. 2018 May;58:47–51.
24. Spatola M, Dalmau J. Seizures and risk of epilepsy in autoimmune and other inflammatory encephalitis. Curr. Opin. Neurol. 2017 June;30:345–353.
25. Sotgiu S, Murrighile MR, Constantin G. Treatment of refractory epilepsy with natalizumab in a patient with multiple sclerosis. Case report. BMC Neurol. 2010 September 23;10:84.
26. Mahamud Z, Burman J, Zelano J. Risk of epilepsy after a single seizure in multiple sclerosis. Eur. J. Neurol. 2018 June;25:854–860.
27. Bien CG, Holtkamp M. "Autoimmune epilepsy": encephalitis with autoantibodies for epileptologists epilepsy currents. Am. Epilepsy Soc. 2017 May–June;17:134–141.
28. Graus F, Titulaer MJ, Balu R, Benseler S, Bien CG, Cellucci T, et al. A clinical approach to diagnosis of autoimmune encephalitis. Lancet Neurol. 2016 April;15:391–404.
29. Cabezudo-García P, Mena-Vázquez N, Villagrán-García M, Serrano-Castro PJ. Efficacy of anti-epileptic drugs in autoimmune epilepsy: a systematic review. Seizure. 2018;59:72–76. Review.
30. Dittrich TD, Baumann SM, Semmlack S, De Marchis GM, Hunziker S, Ruegg S, et al. Diagnostic yield of cerebrospinal fluid analysis in status epilepticus: an 8-year cohort study. J. Neurol. 2021 September;268:3325–3336.
31. Li Y, Tymchuk S, Barry J, Muppidi S, Le S. Antibody prevalence in epilepsy before surgery (APES) in drug-resistant focal epilepsy. Epilepsia. 2021 January 19;62:720–728.

32. Dubey D, Alqallaf A, Hays R, Freeman M, Chen K, Ding K, et al. Neurological autoantibody prevalence in epilepsy of unknown etiology. JAMA Neurol. 2017 April 1;74:397–402.
33. Jehi L. Searching for autoimmune epilepsy: why, where, and when? epilepsy currents. Am. Epilepsy Soc. 2017 November–December;17:363–364.
34. Dubey D, Singh J, Britton JW, Pittock SJ, Flanagan EP, Lennon VA, et al. Predictive models in the diagnosis and treatment of autoimmune epilepsy. Epilepsia. 2017 July;58:1181–1189.
35. Baumgartner T, Carreno M, Rocamora R, Bisulli F, Boni A, Brazdil M, et al. A survey of the European Reference Network EpiCARE on clinical practice for selected rare epilepsies. Epilepsia Open. 2021 March;6:160–170.
36. Costagliola G, Depietri G, Michev A, Riva A, Foiadelli T, Savasta S, et al. Targeting inflammatory mediators in epilepsy: a systematic review of its molecular basis and clinical applications. Front. Neurol. 2022;13:741244.
37. Ruegg S. Antineuronal antibodies and epilepsy: treat the patient, not the lab. J. Neurol. Neurosurg. Psychiatry. 2021 March;92:230.
38. Dubey D, Britton J, McKeon A, Gadoth A, Zekeridou A, Lopez Chiriboga SA, et al. Randomized placebo-controlled trial of intravenous immunoglobulin in autoimmune LGI1/CASPR2 epilepsy. Ann. Neurol. 2020 February;87:313–323.
39. Kimizu T, Takahashi Y, Oboshi T, Horino A, Omatsu H, Koike T, et al. Methylprednisolone pulse therapy in 31 patients with refractory epilepsy: a single-center retrospective analysis. Epilepsy Behav. 2020 August;109:107116.
40. von Rhein B, Wagner J, Widman G, Malter MP, Elger CE, Helmstaedter C. Suspected antibody negative autoimmune limbic encephalitis: outcome of immunotherapy. Acta Neurol. Scand. 2017 January;135:134–141.
41. Toledano M, Britton JW, McKeon A, Shin C, Lennon VA, Quek AM, et al. Utility of an immunotherapy trial in evaluating patients with presumed autoimmune epilepsy. Neurology. 2014 May 6;82:1578–1586.
42. Uribe-San-Martin R, Ciampi E, Santibanez R, Irani SR, Marquez A, Cruz JP, et al. LGI1-antibody associated epilepsy successfully treated in the outpatient setting. J. Neuroimmunol. 2020 August 15;345:577268.
43. Feyissa AM, Lopez Chiriboga AS, Britton JW. Antiepileptic drug therapy in patients with autoimmune epilepsy. Neurol. Neuroimmunol. Neuroinflamm. 2017 July;4:e353.
44. Rada A, Birnbacher R, Gobbi C, Kurthen M, Ludolph A, Naumann M, et al. Seizures associated with antibodies against cell surface antigens are acute symptomatic and not indicative of epilepsy: insights from long-term data. J. Neurol. 2021 March;268:1059–1069.
45. Melzer N, Rosenow F. Autoimmune-associated epilepsy —a challenging concept. Seizure. 2024 May 27. doi: 10.1016/j.seizure.2024.05.017 (online ahead of print)
46. Wickstrom R, Taraschenko O, Dilena R, Payne ET, Specchio N, Nabbout R, et al. International consensus recommendations for management of new onset refractory status epilepticus (NORSE) incl. febrile infection-related epilepsy syndrome (FIRES): statements and supporting evidence. Epilepsia. 2022 August 23;63:2840–2864.
47. Wesselingh R, Broadley J, Buzzard K, Tarlinton D, Seneviratne U, Kyndt C, et al. Prevalence, risk factors, and prognosis of drug-resistant epilepsy in autoimmune encephalitis. Epilepsy Behav. 2022 July;132:108729.
48. Mahamud Z, Burman J, Zelano J. Prognostic impact of epilepsy in multiple sclerosis. Mult. Scler. Relat. Disord. 2019 November 5;38:101497.
49. Mahadeen AZ, Carlson AK, Cohen JA, Galioto R, Abbatemarco JR, Kunchok A. Review of the longitudinal management of autoimmune encephalitis, potential biomarkers, and novel therapeutics. Neurol. Clin. Pract. 2024 August;14:e200306.
50. Mahamud Z, Hakansson S, Burman J, Zelano J. Retention of antiseizure medications for epilepsy in multiple sclerosis: A retrospective observational study. Epilepsy Behav. 2021 August;121:108034.

Epilepsy in Dementia 6

6.1 RISK OF EPILEPSY

Assessing the risk of epilepsy in dementia is complicated. Both prevalence and incidence estimates vary substantially, and as the European Academy of Neurology guidelines point out, it is not clear how common the entity is.[1] The difficulties facing researchers in establishing prevalence and incidence include subtle seizures being overlooked and that patients are often cared for outside of epilepsy care providers, where there may be less emphasis on diagnosing epilepsy. Establishing etiology in an older population is also difficult—epilepsy becomes more common with advancing age and so do competing epilepsy causes.[2] At least one third of dementia patients with epilepsy have structural abnormalities on brain imaging that offer alternative explanations for their seizures, most commonly vascular lesions.[3] Against this background, the literature is expectedly heterogeneous.

6.1.1 Prevalence

The setting of studies is important when considering prevalence, which was seven times higher in older persons in nursing homes compared to age-matched controls in a US investigation.[4] One UK memory clinic reported that 25% of patients had epilepsy,[5] but other memory clinics can report lower rates at about 3%.[6] In epilepsy cohorts, dementia seems much rarer. In a tertiary epilepsy center in Germany, only 0.25% had dementia.[7]

Population-based investigations also vary in their estimates. Only 4% of patients in the Swedish dementia register had or developed epilepsy.[8] Conversely, among patients over 70 with epilepsy in rural Pennsylvania, 18% had dementia.[9] Of course, cognitive impairment that does not qualify as dementia is quite common in epilepsy and reported in 48% of patients at epilepsy clinics in one study.[10]

6.1.2 Incidence

Dementia increases the risk of epilepsy but is still rarely encountered in epilepsy practice compared to other causes. The general health of the studied population including vascular risk factors are probably of importance also in incidence studies. Out of first seizures in the US or Sweden, only about 2% were attributed to

DOI: 10.1201/9781003501404-6

dementia,[11,12] whereas in China, 7% of new-onset epilepsy in patients over 60 was classified as caused by dementia.[13] In US veterans, dementia increases the risk of new-onset epilepsy four-fold,[14] but patients in the national Swedish dementia register had only a 2.5-fold increased risk of epilepsy after the dementia diagnosis compared to age-matched controls.[8] The Swedish rate is close to findings in the US Framingham study of a general population sample, in which dementia entailed a two-fold increased risk of developing epilepsy.[15] An approximate two- to three-fold increased risk of epilepsy after a diagnosis of dementia is probably a reasonable estimate in industrialized countries.

There is an ongoing discussion about whether late-onset epilepsy increases the risk of dementia, with cumulative long-term risks of 17%–40% in some studies.[16,17] The risk of dementia in patients with epilepsy was increased two- to three-fold in large US studies,[15,18] but causality is difficult to establish. Several other factors than the epilepsy *per se* could increase the risk of dementia—like underlying neurodegeneration, antiseizure medications, and shared vascular risk factors.

6.1.2.1 Alzheimer's Disease and Vascular Dementia

Alzheimer's disease and vascular dementia are often discussed as particularly prone to cause epilepsy. Reported seizure prevalences in Alzheimer's disease range from 1.5% to 64%,[19] with a study of neuropathologically verified Alzheimer's reporting that 17% (11/64) of patients had epilepsy.[20] Patients with Alzheimer's disease have an increased risk of first unprovoked seizures compared to similar age groups without dementia.[21] Another study found that 4.7% of patients with Alzheimer's developed epilepsy, resulting in an adjusted HR of 1.85 (1.20–2.83).[22] In a UK primary care study, patients with Alzheimer's disease or vascular dementia had an incidence rate of epilepsy that was seven to nine times greater than that of a control group.[23] This is high compared to a Finish register-based study, in which 2.1% of patients with

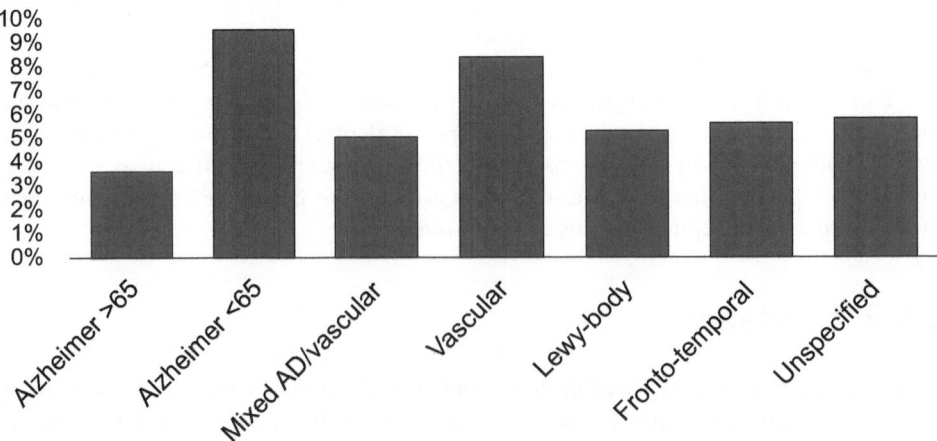

FIGURE 6.1 Cumulative incidence of epilepsy or seizure in patients in the Swedish dementia register by clinical dementia diagnosis.[8]

Alzheimer's disease had epilepsy, resulting in an OR of 1.66 compared to the general population of the same age.[24]

6.2 EPILEPSY IN RARER DEMENTIA FORMS

In addition to the larger groups of neurodegenerative dementias, there are some rare forms sometimes encountered in general neurology.

6.2.1 Late-Onset Myoclonic Epilepsy in Down Syndrome

Down syndrome is a genetic neurodegenerative condition in which Alzheimer's-like dementia is a frequent complication after 50 years of age. The prevalence of epilepsy in Down syndrome is high, but the characteristics of the epilepsy seem to vary with the age of onset. One relatively large series described seizures in a quarter of patients over 50 years of age.[25] In late-onset epilepsy, a myoclonic type of generalized epilepsy predominates and has been suggested to share pathophysiological mechanisms with the myoclonic epilepsy seen in Alzheimer's disease.[26] Some treatment options mentioned in the literature include levetiracetam, piracetam, valproate, and topiramate.[26,27] There is little robust evidence and trials with registered ASMs based on clinical judgment of what suits each patient is probably best.

6.2.2 Huntington's Disease

One large multicenter study detected epilepsy in 38% of juvenile patients with Huntington's disease.[28] The main risk factor was the young age at onset. The most common seizure types were tonic-clonic seizures, followed by tonic, myoclonic seizures, and staring spells. Multiple seizure types were not uncommon. The efficacy of different ASMs was not clear from the report. In patients with adult-onset Huntington's disease, epilepsy was present in three patients, constituting just 2.6% (0.6%–7.5%) of a Finish cohort. Tonic-clonic seizures were the most common type. Patients developed epilepsy with onset age 33–56 and the epilepsy seemed well controlled with the first ASM (carbamazepine or valproate) in monotherapy.[29]

6.2.3 Creutzfeldt–Jakob Disease

Seizures have been reported in 40% of some study populations with sporadic Creutzfeldt–Jakob disease, but typical estimates range from a few percent at onset rising to around 15% during the disease course.[30] The risk of seizures seems somewhat lower in familial forms of CJD than sporadic disease, but the relative rarity prevents any firm conclusions.[31] In patients with rapidly progressive encephalopathy, non-convulsive status epilepticus can be a contributor to the clinical picture and treatment of status epilepticus helpful.[32,33] There is however a discussion on whether the EEG changes interpreted as non-convulsive SE are in fact an epiphenomena of the prion pathology rather than actual status epilepticus.

6.3 EPILEPTOGENESIS

Epileptogenesis in dementia is poorly understood, and mechanisms probably vary with the dementia type. Possible mechanisms include hyperexcitability by plaques or disruption of brain networks through neuronal loss. In vascular or other subcortical dementias, structural disruption of networks can probably result in epilepsy.

Clinically, there is often a temporal relationship between epilepsy and dementia suggesting that neurodegeneration plays a role in epileptogenesis. For patients in the Swedish dementia register diagnosed with epilepsy, onset was often in the decade spanning the dementia diagnosis.[8] Similarly, 12 (6.8%) out of 177 patients with new-onset seizures at a memory clinic in Liverpool had epilepsy, and seven of these had onset of seizures roughly corresponding to the onset of cognitive symptoms.[34] The average latency from Alzheimer's diagnosis to seizure onset in patients with epilepsy was 3.6 years in one investigation,[22] which fits well with the Swedish register data.

Alzheimer's disease is particularly interesting because of the relatively high clinical risk of epilepsy compared to many other dementias. Different plausible mechanisms have been found, including direct effects of amyloid-ß, tau, selective dysfunction of certain interneurons, astrocyte and microglia dysfunction, ApoE4, neurovascular unit dysfunction, and sleep disturbance.[35] In a human familial form of Alzheimer's disease, epilepsy is a relatively common and early feature.[36] Nonetheless, only about one third of patients with presenilin-2 mutations have seizures, so the phenotype seems variable and much remains to be understood.[36] Mouse models of Alzheimer's, like presenilin-2 knock-out mice, demonstrate high frequency oscillations on EEG, which are considered relatively specific for epilepsy.[37] Regarding amyloid-ß, familial Alzheimer's mouse models show that a high level of plaque deposition is associated with increased susceptibility to chemoconvulsants.[38] Amyloid dynamics and production are regulated by neuronal activity,[39] which could explain the relationship between plaques and seizures. Chemically induced seizures result in accelerated accumulation of plaques in mice.[40]

Recently, indications have emerged that similar processes are important in humans, particularly a bidirectional association between Alzheimer's disease and seizures. Patients with Alzheimer's and patients with epilepsy have similarities in proteomic expression.[41] A large drop in the blood $A\beta_{42}/A\beta_{40}$ ratio from midlife to later life (a low ratio is believed to reflect plaque deposition in the brain and increases the risk of Alzheimer's disease) is associated with an increased risk of later epilepsy.[42] The neuronal protein tau is deposited in many dementias, including Alzheimer's disease, and could also play a pathophysiological role. Tau is sometimes found in increased levels in some epileptic tissue removed in epilepsy surgery, and animal models of dementia with tau pathology show epilepsy phenotypes.[43,44]

Myoclonia can develop in the final stages of many dementias. It is not clear if this reflects specific disease mechanisms involved in myoclonia in other epilepsies or a final common pathway of extensive neurodegeneration.

In summary, many different mechanisms could contribute to epilepsy in patients with dementia. It is important to stress that many mechanisms are possible and even plausible causal factors, but the field so far struggles to understand the large clinical variability. In very advanced Alzheimer's disease, many patients could have at least subclinical seizures, but why do not all patients with Alzheimer's get epilepsy? Researchers have yet to find good ways to track and interfere with the neuropathological pathways discussed earlier for a better understanding. For instance, it will be interesting to see if the new Alzheimer's disease treatments with plaque-targeting antibodies will reduce the rates of epilepsy.

6.3.1 Biomarkers

Biomarkers of Alzheimer's disease have developed rapidly in the last decade, but so far this has not translated into clinically useful tools that can detect epileptogenesis. Some studies suggest that more pronounced Alzheimer's pathology is linked to epilepsy. For instance, a large study on Swedish patients that had undergone examination of cerebrospinal fluid as part of a dementia work-up found that those developing epilepsy had more pronounced Alzheimer's pathology.[45] Concentrations of total tau and phosphorylated tau were higher in patients with epilepsy than the levels in patients without epilepsy, and amyloid beta 42 levels were significantly lower in Alzheimer's disease patients with epilepsy. There were no differences in the concentration of brain injury markers like neurofilament or glial fibrillary acidic protein, suggesting that the differences were a reflection of Alzheimer's pathology rather than more advanced neurodegeneration. The study again underlines the close link between Alzheimer's pathology and epilepsy.

6.4 RISK FACTORS

Dementia type seems to be an important clinical risk factor with regards to epilepsy. Alzheimer's disease was associated with an odds ratio of hospitalization for epilepsy of 3.07 (2.98–3.16) in US patients over age 55, compared to 2.21 (2.14–2.27) for non-Alzheimer's dementia.[46] In the Swedish dementia register, early-onset Alzheimer's disease was one of the dementia types with the highest risk of epilepsy or seizures (Figure 6.1),[8] in agreement with other studies.[21] Higher cumulative incidences have been reported in other studies, like 13% in Alzheimer's, 14% in dementia with Lewy bodies, and 3% in frontal lobe dementia.[47] Underdiagnosis of epilepsy in routine care and reliance on clinical categorization of dementias are likely to explain some of the differences.

Dementia severity is another risk factor (Table 6.1). Most studies find that low Mini-Mental State Examination (MMSE) score or other indicators of dementia severity is a risk factor for epilepsy. This was the case for patients in the Swedish dementia register as well as in a study on patients with vascular dementia and Alzheimer's.[23] Interestingly, the latter study found disease duration to be a risk factor for epilepsy only in Alzheimer's and not in vascular dementia, which perhaps indicates the pathogenic role of accumulated Alzheimer's pathology as opposed to the more stepwise disease process in vascular dementia.

6.4.1 Risk of Recurrence after a First Unprovoked Seizure

Four studies have reported quite different recurrence risks after a first seizure in dementia—probably because of variations in inclusion criteria. One is a retrospective review of autopsy-verified Alzheimer's disease, in which 69% of 77 patients had more than one seizure, but only 29% had more than two seizures. The authors specified, "The typical patient was institutionalized, had severe memory loss, was unable to solve problems, had little independent function, and required a great deal of assistance in activities of daily living."[48] The second is a prospective study of persons with Alzheimer's disease that found a recurrence risk of 29%, but it had just 14 participants and short follow-up.[49] Young age, epileptiform discharges, and severe cognitive symptoms were risk factors for seizure recurrence in one study of Alzheimer's disease.[50]

In a large register-based (not population-wide) study in Sweden, we found a 32% survival-adjusted risk of epilepsy five years after a first seizure. The study was based on all patients in the Swedish dementia register, which may have an overrepresentation of patients seen at specialized centers (probably young and severe patients).[51] Subgroups with higher risks were patients with dementia onset <70 years of age (48% developed epilepsy), and early-onset Alzheimer's disease (50% developed epilepsy).[51] An often cited study on seizure recurrence in Alzheimer's reports a seizure recurrence risk of 70%, but it is not a first seizure study.[52]

TABLE 6.1   Risk Factors of Epilepsy in Dementia[8]

Young age
Male sex
Stroke, head trauma, and brain tumor
Dementia type (vascular and young-onset Alzheimer's have high risk)
Low MMSE score

CASE 6.1 First Seizure in New-Onset Dementia

A 62-year-old man is seen in the seizure clinic after a first seizure. He has recently been diagnosed with minimal cognitive impairment and has a CSF profile in keeping with a diagnosis of Alzheimer's disease. The work up with EEG and MRI is unremarkable.

Comment: At the moment, there is insufficient evidence to estimate a precise recurrence risk in this patient. The risk is probably slightly elevated because of the neurodegenerative disease, but not certainly at the threshold for an epilepsy diagnosis.

6.5 MANAGEMENT

6.5.1 Clinical Presentation

6.5.1.1 Seizures

There are challenges in diagnosing epilepsy in patients with dementia. Apart from assessment of seizure recurrence risk, recognition of seizures as well as exclusion of differential diagnoses are key elements that can take some time. A good history, careful follow-up, and avoiding too rapid conclusions is often helpful.

Regarding recognition of seizures, patients may be unable to give adequate description of their symptoms, live alone, and have a semiology different from that of younger patients. Convulsions are typically more rare than in younger persons with epilepsy.[5,53–55] Many studies suggest that new-onset epilepsy in patients with dementia often entails focal subtle seizures causing impaired awareness alone,[3,47] although tonic-clonic seizures can occur.[56] The proportions of different seizure types were studied in a large UK project on many forms of dementia, which found new-onset seizures to be focal aware in 7%, focal with impaired awareness in 53%, and tonic-clonic in 40%. During the disease course, 57% of all patients had tonic-clonic seizures and 8% developed myoclonus.[57] Other reports suggest that focal non-motor seizures are the most common, with motor and bilateral tonic-clonic seizures being more rare.[49] Non-motor seizures can have behavioral, cognitive, or sensory symptoms, but behavioral arrest is perhaps most common, and difficult to detect.

Myoclonus is a relatively common seizure type seen in epilepsy in dementia. In one study, the cumulative risk of myoclonus was 60% for patients with dementia with Lewy bodies, 45% for patients with Alzheimer's disease, and 20% for patients with frontotemporal dementia. Since myoclonus is a late feature, the prevalence was lower than the cumulative risk; 27% for dementia with Lewy bodies, 13% for frontotemporal dementia, and 8.5% for Alzheimer's disease.[47] Why myoclonus differs between different dementia forms is not known, but it may reflect relative subcortical network disruption.

An interesting ambulatory EEG study characterized seizures in patients with Alzheimer's disease. Out of 42 patients, 24% had seizures. The majority were focal aware seizures without motor activity. Subclinical epileptiform discharges were found in 28%. Long-term EEG monitoring was suggested as a means to increase yield and diagnostic accuracy.[58]

THE VALUE OF EEG

Standard EEG has been reported to be less sensitive in older patients, but video-EEG may be a good option and is probably underutilized.[53] Epileptiform discharges are found in 16%–38% of patients with epilepsy in different forms of dementia, but whether this represents epilepsy (a predisposition for unprovoked seizures) is hard to know.[3,21] In a UK study of patients with epilepsy and dementia, 23%–31% of patients had epileptiform activity on their first EEG.[57] Up to 42% of Alzheimer's patients have epileptiform activity on EEG.[59] Another illustrative EEG study of an unselected memory clinic population found epileptiform activity in 3%, 60% of whom did not have seizures. In patients without an epilepsy diagnosis at the time of their EEG, only 20% of patients with positive EEG and a dementia diagnosis had a subsequent unprovoked seizure.[60]

In summary, EEG can be useful to determine if certain episodes are caused by epilepsy—but it is not suitable as a screening tool. Clinical judgment is important to avoid overinterpretation of negative results as well as the significance of epileptiform activity.

6.5.2 Estimating Recurrence Risk after a First Seizure

Translating the very sparse literature on risks of seizure into clinical practice is not uncomplicated. Some risk estimates are provided in Figure 6.2, but these are based on administrative data and relatively crude. The most important clinical insight is that a diagnosis of dementia does not automatically mean that a first seizure mandates a diagnosis of epilepsy and treatment. That being said, recurrence risks are probably higher than in patients without a brain disorder. To further complicate the matter of when to start treatment, seizures are often relatively mild with regards to semiology, survival is often limited, and patients are often supervised, making seizure-related risks lower. Being older, patients can also be more sensitive to side effects.

Clinical judgment and involvement of the patient and carers is key in establishing a good treatment plan. Sometimes treatment is motivated after a first seizure, but more often it is better to await recurrence before starting ASM therapy which is likely to be life-long. On the other hand, several studies have made it plausible that a subset of patients

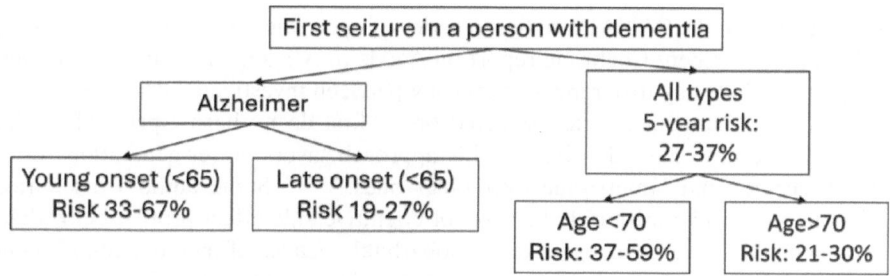

FIGURE 6.2   Risk of epilepsy after a first seizure in patients with dementia.

with seizures in dementia have cognitive symptoms that can be improved with treatment. A good history and careful witness description in search of subclinical seizures are probably the best method for identification of such cases at the moment. Several studies on Alzheimer's cohorts with suspected or diagnosed epilepsy report relatively high rates of untreated patients.[49] This would be rare in other epilepsy populations and illustrates that clinicians are aware of the delicate balance between over- and undertreatment with ASMs.

6.5.3 Detecting Dementia in New-Onset Epilepsy

The insidious onset of neurodegenerative disorders means that patients can sometimes present with relatively preserved cognitive functions after a first seizure, but then develop more and more signs of dementia. Some of these cases may be coincidental occurrences, but as discussed earlier there is an overrepresentation of epilepsy diagnoses in the five years proceeding a diagnosis of dementia. Detection of dementia can sometimes be delayed because dysexecutive symptoms, memory problems, and emotional instability can be mistaken for ASM side effects or reactions to the epilepsy diagnosis itself. Clinical vigilance and use of supporting tests like dementia markers in CSF or atrophy patterns on imaging, neuropsychological testing, and follow-up can often help. If a dementia diagnosis can be detected in time, it can often help both the patient and their family to get access to adequate treatment, support, and better prognostic information.

6.6 TREATMENT

6.6.1 Medical Treatment of Epilepsy

As can be expected for a heterogeneous patient population dispersed throughout most healthcare systems and unable to consent to research, there is little longitudinal randomized data on the efficacy of ASM treatment of epilepsy in Alzheimer's disease, and no good data for rarer forms of dementia. For instance, persons with known dementia were excluded from the SANAD studies, a series of open randomized trials comparing several ASMs.[61] A recent Cochrane report on ASMs in Alzheimer's found insufficient evidence to conclude any differences in efficacy between investigated drugs.[62]

In practice, treatment is often selected on a "first do no harm" principle, using drugs that cause minimal side effects. This approach favors newer-generation ASMs like levetiracetam and lamotrigine over older ones.[35,63–65] Some authors discourage use of topiramate and zonisamide because of cognitive side effect profile, benzodiazepines or other GABAergic drugs like phenobarbital because of memory impairment, falls, and high frequency of side effects, carbamazepine and phenytoin because of poor tolerability in the elderly, and valproic acid because of encephalopathic potential.[35,65] Overall, these are expert opinions, and clinical care must be based on clinical judgment. Some authors argue that lamotrigine should be preferred over levetiracetam, because of the better side effect profile and better effectiveness demonstrated in SANAD II.[61]

It is probably wise to tailor the ASM choice to patient characteristics and to avoid ASMs that can interfere with other medications or aggravate behavioral or medical problems. Importantly, the goal is not only to prevent seizures, but also to overall improve quality of life. In this regard, overtreatment as well as undertreatment of epilepsy can cause problems. An overall perspective and careful follow-up including enquiring about both side effects and subtle seizure symptoms may be required to strike the right balance. ASM doses should often start low and be titrated according to response to avoid unnecessary side effects. Lower doses also often work well in older patients with regards to seizure suppression, for unknown reasons.

6.6.1.1 Choosing the Right ASM

Levetiracetam and lamotrigine are discussed as having a better side effect profile than older ASMs in the European Academy guidelines for treatment of epilepsy in dementia.[1] These ASMs were indeed better tolerated than phenytoin in epilepsy in a study on early-stage Alzheimer's disease,[85] and levetiracetam was better tolerated than both lamotrigine and phenobarbital in another study on patients with Alzheimer's disease.[66] Hopefully, this is being implemented in routine clinical care. Levetiracetam was the most common ASM in a large study of patients with epilepsy at a dementia clinic in the UK and used in 54%.[57] In a Swedish population-based study on prescription data evaluating continued treatment (retention) as an integrated measure of effect and tolerability, levetiracetam was also the most common choice. Lamotrigine and levetiracetam also had higher retention rates than carbamazepine.[67] These results agree with smaller uncontrolled prospective studies,[68] suggesting that levetiracetam or lamotrigine are currently often reasonable first options.

The reports of increasing use of newer-generation ASMs are not unequivocal. There are also several reports indicating an unfortunately high use of older-generation ASMs in patients with dementia. For instance, a study on patients with Alzheimer's disease in Finland found a higher use of older-generation ASMs than in non-Alzheimer's patients.[24] If patients with older ASMs should be switched to newer variants with milder side effects and a more beneficial profile with regards to drug–drug interactions is often a difficult clinical question. The standard rule is not to interfere with an epilepsy treatment that is working, but on the other hand there is sometimes much to be gained if tiredness or memory problems can be reduced. Clinical judgment is currently the best guide, as is the involvement of the patient and caregivers in deciding the appropriate course of action.

6.6.1.2 Revise Therapy If Needed

In general epilepsy populations, only about half of patients will do well on the first ASM they try. There is little reason to believe that epilepsy in dementia is markedly different. Side effects are the main cause of therapy revision in cognitively competent persons, but these may be more difficult to detect in persons with dementia. Vigilance for tiredness, altered mood, or behavioral problems and switching an ASM if needed can sometimes have dramatic effects. It is important to keep in mind that the overall aim is quality of life, not merely seizure freedom.

CASE 6.2 Starting and Revising ASM Therapy

An 82-year-old woman with Alzheimer's dementia is referred because of staring spells and chewing movements of the mouth that occur about monthly. They last about 20 seconds and do not seem to bother her or affect quality of life. She lives in a nursing home. Focal epilepsy is diagnosed, but ASM is not started. After two months, the patient has a tonic-clonic seizure and is started on a first ASM. Despite a low dose, she has extensive tiredness and is switched to a different ASM. There are no more seizures and QoL seems good.

Comment: The case illustrates the intricacies of starting ASM therapy or not. Treatment in older patients is very likely to cause side effects (which indeed turned out to be the case). On the other hand, the patient had a tonic-clonic seizure which may not have happened had the smaller seizures been treated. Clinical judgment and patient/caregiver opinion must decide on the best course of action in each case. Vigilance regarding side effects and revision of therapy as needed is important.

6.6.1.3 Withdrawal

There are no firm guidelines on withdrawal of ASMs in patients with epilepsy in dementia. In general, because it is a progressive disease, the predisposition for seizures is unlikely to subside. However, side effects and the ever-present risk that non-epileptic paroxysmal events may have been misdiagnosed as seizures makes it difficult to say that withdrawal of ASM therapy should never be attempted. In suspected cases of ASM-induced cognitive problems or encephalopathy, withdrawal of therapy and close clinical monitoring can be necessary. Patients or caregivers considering stopping ASM should be advised that a longer period of seizure freedom (many years) is recommended before attempting to withdraw therapy, that consequences of seizure recurrence need to be carefully considered beforehand, that the risks of seizure recurrence are difficult to estimate, and that the effectiveness of a restarted therapy cannot be guaranteed.

6.6.1.4 Treatment of Other Symptoms than Seizures

ASMs are sometimes used for indications other than epilepsy, and results from those studies provide interesting information on side effect profiles of the drugs when used in the dementia population. Valproate was for instance not well tolerated in a study of patients with Alzheimer's disease (used for behavioral clinical symptoms).[69] Valproate encephalopathy is a very important clinical entity characterized mainly by reduced consciousness. Seizures may worsen. Ammonium levels are sometimes, but not always, elevated. Parkinsonian features can be an important diagnostic clue and early warning sign.[70] Lamotrigine has been evaluated in small studies for treatment of behavioral problems in dementia and also for cognition, with favorable results in small patient materials.[71]

There is currently renewed interest in whether subclinical seizure activity may contribute to cognitive symptoms in Alzheimer's disease.[72,73] In patients with cognitive impairment and interictal epileptiform activity, administration of antiepileptic drugs improved cognition slightly in one study.[74] Transient epileptic amnesia is a special type of cognitive seizure that has been suggested to cause some wandering behavioral symptoms in Alzheimer's disease.[56] The same phenomenon has also been reported to precede Alzheimer's in a case report.[75] One study reported that patients with Alzheimer's disease that had subclinical epileptiform activity showed faster cognitive decline than patients without epileptiform activity.[59] Recently, a post hoc analysis of a levetiracetam trial in Alzheimer's disease found that in patients with epileptiform activity, a few cognitive outcomes were improved during treatment.[76] This echoes some previous reports from earlier studies that ASMs can improve cognitive performance in patients with epilepsy and Alzheimer's disease.[66] That treatment of seizures improves cognition is not very surprising, but the interesting question is if treatment with ASMs has a value also in patients without overt seizures. More studies of levetiracetam and perhaps other ASMs for cognitive outcomes in Alzheimer's disease are likely to follow.

DO ANTISEIZURE MEDICATIONS CAUSE DEMENTIA?

An interesting discussion is whether ASMs increase the risk of dementia. This has been suggested based on statistical associations, but since onset of epilepsy may precede cognitive decline by many years, an underlying dementia disorder may potentially have confounded the analysis.[77,78] There are also suggestions that cognitive impairment may proceed faster in patients with epilepsy and other brain diseases; an entity called accelerated cognitive decline.[79] Risk factors of this phenomenon, which may occur in patients with or without dementia, are brain comorbidity, low educational level, and older age.[80] Suspicion of valproate encephalopathy is important. Future studies on risks of dementia in users of different ASMs are likely to inform the matter.

6.6.2 Non-Medical Treatments

Epilepsy surgery and VNS therapy have not been systematically evaluated in patients with dementia.[54]

6.7 PROGNOSIS

6.7.1 Seizures

Large prospective cohort studies on the prognosis of epilepsy in dementia have not been done, so many questions remain regarding seizure freedom and retention rates of different antiepileptic drugs.[53] Smaller studies report highly varying rates of seizure freedom, from 79% being seizure free to only 27%.[3,66] Pharmacoresistance is rarely reported as an outcome, so whether the proportion of patients not responding to treatment is different from that of other epilepsy populations is unclear. A recurring theme in many studies is that relatively few patients have a high seizure frequency, at least of detectable seizures. In 27 patients with Alzheimer's that were followed for a year, only eight reported having seizures during a 12-month follow-up, and only four had been on ASMs.[49] Older reports of large cohorts of dementia inpatients report somewhat higher rates, in one study reaching over two seizures per patient and year, but the dementia was probably more severe.[81] There is a lack of studies on risk factors for pharmacoresistance.

In keeping with high seizure frequency being relatively rare, investigations on status epilepticus have not indicated that patients with dementia are at a particularly high risk. A Swedish register-based investigation found dementia to be the etiology least likely to be associated with status epilepticus (36/100.000 person years) compared to stroke or brain infections (64/100.000 person years). Overall, only 0.1% of patients with dementia had status epilepticus. If only patients with diagnoses of both epilepsy and dementia were considered, the incidence of SE was naturally much higher (354/100.000 person years), but still about half that of persons with epilepsy after stroke.[82] On the other hand, patients with dementia and one or two other brain comorbidities had higher risk of status epilepticus.

6.7.2 Cognition

The cognitive decline is usually more pronounced in persons with epilepsy and dementia than in persons with only dementia. It is difficult to assess if this reflects an interaction between epilepsy and dementia or an additive effect of epilepsy and seizures on preexisting cognitive problems caused by the dementia. An ambitious investigation of persons with Alzheimer's disease with and without epilepsy demonstrated that cognitive problems were more common at baseline, but also that the gap between epilepsy

TABLE 6.2   Clinical Take-Home Messages

- Approximately 4% of persons with dementia will be diagnosed with epilepsy.
- Young-onset Alzheimer's and vascular dementia are subtypes with high risk.
- Epilepsy often arises in a time span from five years before to five years after the onset of dementia.
- Clinically, seizures may be subtle and underrecognized.
- The aim of antiseizure medication therapy is quality of life; absence of all symptoms suspected to be seizures may not be worth the side effects.
- A first seizure in a person with dementia may not indicate a high recurrence risk motivating diagnosis of epilepsy. Whether therapy is motivated depends on each case—the severity of the seizure and individual risk of recurrence.
- Epileptiform activity on EEG may occur without a patient ever having a seizure.
- Newer generation antiseizure medications like lamotrigine and levetiracetam are often recommended because of a milder side effect profile than previous generations. There is very little high-level evidence.

and non-epilepsy patients widened during the follow-up time of 12 months.[49] Attention, verbal fluency, problem solving, and personal care were particularly affected. For other non-seizure outcomes, dementia is a risk factor for not living independently in older patients with epilepsy.[9]

6.7.3 Survival

Compared to many other forms of epilepsy, the mortality in dementia patients with epilepsy is high.[8] This probably reflects a relatively severe dementia and that epilepsy ensues as a late symptom. In a long-term follow-up of patients in the Swedish dementia register, the mean survival time after a first seizure was less than three years.[51] Whether epilepsy contributed to the deaths is difficult to study—postmortem examinations of older patients may not always be extensive and epilepsy-related causes of death are often overlooked. Dementia is a common comorbidity in diseased persons with epilepsy,[83] but this may simply reflect the high mortality of dementia. Detailed analysis of expert-assessed SUDEP cases have not identified dementia as a particular risk factor for SUDEP.[84] Clinical take home messages are presented in Table 6.2.

REFERENCES

1. Frederiksen KS, Cooper C, Frisoni GB, Frolich L, Georges J, Kramberger MG, et al. A European Academy of Neurology guideline on medical management issues in dementia. Eur. J. Neurol. 2020 October;27:1805–1820.
2. Beghi E, Giussani G. Aging and the epidemiology of epilepsy. Neuroepidemiology. 2018;51:216–223.

3. Rao SC, Dove G, Cascino GD, Petersen RC. Recurrent seizures in patients with dementia: frequency, seizure types, and treatment outcome. Epilepsy Behav. 2009 January;14:118–120.
4. Birnbaum AK, Leppik IE, Svensden K, Eberly LE. Prevalence of epilepsy/seizures as a comorbidity of neurologic disorders in nursing homes. Neurology. 2017 February 21;88:750–757.
5. Baker J, Libretto T, Henley W, Zeman A. The prevalence and clinical features of epileptic seizures in a memory clinic population. Seizure. 2019 October;71:83–92.
6. Giorgi FS, Baldacci F, Dini E, Tognoni G, Bonuccelli U. Epilepsy occurrence in patients with Alzheimer's disease: clinical experience in a tertiary dementia center. Neurol. Sci. 2016 April;37:645–647.
7. Helmstaedter C, Lutz T, Wolf V, Witt JA. Prevalence of dementia in a level 4 university epilepsy center: how big is the problem? Front. Neurol. 2023;14:1217594.
8. Zelano J, Brigo F, Garcia-Patek S. Increased risk of epilepsy in patients registered in the Swedish Dementia Registry. Eur. J. Neurol. 2020 January;27:129–135.
9. Baran M, Stecker MM. Epilepsy in a rural elderly population. Epileptic. Disord. 2007 September;9:256–270.
10. Aji BM, Larner AJ. Cognitive assessment in an epilepsy clinic using the AD8 questionnaire. Epilepsy Behav. 2018 August;85:234–236.
11. Ruggles KH, Haessly SM, Berg RL. Prospective study of seizures in the elderly in the Marshfield Epidemiologic Study Area (MESA). Epilepsia. 2001 December;42:1594–1599.
12. Adelow C, Andell E, Amark P, Andersson T, Hellebro E, Ahlbom A, et al. Newly diagnosed single unprovoked seizures and epilepsy in Stockholm, Sweden: first report from the Stockholm Incidence Registry of Epilepsy (SIRE). Epilepsia. 2009 May;50:1094–1101.
13. Guo Y, Yu L, He B, Li S, Zhu Q, Sun H. Aetiological features of elderly patients with newly diagnosed symptomatic epilepsy in western China. Biomed. Res. Int. 2018;2018:4104691.
14. Pugh MJ, Knoefel JE, Mortensen EM, Amuan ME, Berlowitz DR, Van Cott AC. New-onset epilepsy risk factors in older veterans. J. Am. Geriatr. Soc. 2009 February;57:237–242.
15. Stefanidou M, Beiser AS, Himali JJ, Peng TJ, Devinsky O, Seshadri S, et al. The bi-directional association between epilepsy and dementia. The Framingham Heart Study. Neurology. 2020 October 23;95:e3241–e3247.
16. Kawakami O, Koike Y, Ando T, Sugiura M, Kato H, Hiraga K, et al. Incidence of dementia in patients with adult-onset epilepsy of unknown causes. J. Neurol. Sci. 2018 December 15;395:71–76.
17. Costa C, Romoli M, Liguori C, Farotti L, Eusebi P, Bedetti C, et al. Alzheimer's disease and late-onset epilepsy of unknown origin: two faces of beta amyloid pathology. Neurobiol. Aging. 2019 January;73:61–67.
18. Johnson EL, Krauss GL, Kucharska-Newton A, Albert MS, Brandt J, Walker KA, et al. Dementia in late-onset epilepsy: the atherosclerosis risk in communities study. Neurology. 2020 October 23;95:e3248–e3256.
19. Nicastro N, Assal F, Seeck M. From here to epilepsy: the risk of seizure in patients with Alzheimer's disease. Epileptic. Disord. 2016 March;18:1–12.
20. Rauramaa T, Saxlin A, Lohvansuu K, Alafuzoff I, Pitkanen A, Soininen H. Epilepsy in neuropathologically verified Alzheimer's disease. Seizure. 2018 May;58:9–12.
21. Scarmeas N, Honig LS, Choi H, Cantero J, Brandt J, Blacker D, et al. Seizures in Alzheimer disease: who, when, and how common? Arch. Neurol. 2009 August;66:992–997.
22. Cheng CH, Liu CJ, Ou SM, Yeh CM, Chen TJ, Lin YY, et al. Incidence and risk of seizures in Alzheimer's disease: a nationwide population-based cohort study. Epilepsy Res. 2015 September;115:63–66.
23. Imfeld P, Bodmer M, Schuerch M, Jick SS, Meier CR. Seizures in patients with Alzheimer's disease or vascular dementia: a population-based nested case-control analysis. Epilepsia. 2013 April;54:700–707.

24. Bell JS, Lonnroos E, Koivisto AM, Lavikainen P, Laitinen ML, Soininen H, et al. Use of antiepileptic drugs among community-dwelling persons with Alzheimer's disease in Finland. J. Alzheimers Dis. 2011;26:231–237.

25. Real de Asua D, Quero M, Moldenhauer F, Suarez C. Clinical profile and main comorbidities of Spanish adults with Down syndrome. Eur. J. Intern. Med. 2015 July;26:385–391.

26. Moller JC, Hamer HM, Oertel WH, Rosenow F. Late-onset myoclonic epilepsy in Down's syndrome (LOMEDS). Seizure. 2001 June;10:303–306.

27. Sangani M, Shahid A, Amina S, Koubeissi M. Improvement of myoclonic epilepsy in Down syndrome treated with levetiracetam. Epileptic. Disord. 2010 June;12:151–154.

28. Cloud LJ, Rosenblatt A, Margolis RL, Ross CA, Pillai JA, Corey-Bloom J, et al. Seizures in juvenile Huntington's disease: frequency and characterization in a multicenter cohort. Mov. Disord. 2012 December;27:1797–1800.

29. Sipila JO, Soilu-Hanninen M, Majamaa K. Comorbid epilepsy in Finnish patients with adult-onset Huntington's disease. BMC Neurol. 2016 February 10;16:24.

30. Wieser HG, Schindler K, Zumsteg D. EEG in Creutzfeldt–Jakob disease. Clin. Neurophysiol. 2006 May;117:935–951.

31. Appel S, Chapman J, Cohen OS, Rosenmann H, Nitsan Z, Blatt I. Seizures in E200K familial and sporadic Creutzfeldt–Jakob disease. Acta Neurol. Scand. 2015 March;131:152–157.

32. Fanella M, Valente G, Borrello L, Marinelli F, Bracaglia M, Di Marco O, et al. Nonconvulsive status epilepticus versus periodic EEG pattern in sporadic Creutzfeldt–Jakob disease: two sides of the same coin? Int. J. Neurosci. 2024 December;134(12):1606–1610.

33. Srichawla BS. Sporadic Creutzfeldt–Jakob disease with status epilepticus: molecular mechanisms and a scoping review of the literature. Cureus. 2022 August;14:e28649.

34. Lozsadi DA, Larner AJ. Prevalence and causes of seizures at the time of diagnosis of probable Alzheimer's disease. Dement. Geriatr. Cogn. Disord. 2006;22:121–124.

35. Kamondi A, Grigg-Damberger M, Loscher W, Tanila H, Horvath AA. Epilepsy and epileptiform activity in late-onset Alzheimer disease: clinical and pathophysiological advances, gaps and conundrums. Nat. Rev. Neurol. 2024 March;20:162–182.

36. Jayadev S, Leverenz JB, Steinbart E, Stahl J, Klunk W, Yu CE, et al. Alzheimer's disease phenotypes and genotypes associated with mutations in presenilin 2. Brain J. Neurol. 2010 April;133:1143–1154.

37. Lisgaras CP, Scharfman HE. High-frequency oscillations (250 –500 Hz) in animal models of Alzheimer's disease and two animal models of epilepsy. Epilepsia. 2023 January;64:231–246.

38. Born HA. Seizures in Alzheimer's disease. Neuroscience. 2015 February 12;286:251–263.

39. Zou Y, Wang C, Li H, Zhong M, Lin J, Hu Y, et al. Epileptic seizures induced by pentylenetetrazole kindling accelerate Alzheimer-like neuropathology in 5xFAD mice. Front Pharmacol. 2024;15:1500105.

40. Yan XX, Cai Y, Shelton J, Deng SH, Luo XG, Oddo S, et al. Chronic temporal lobe epilepsy is associated with enhanced Alzheimer-like neuropathology in 3xTg-AD mice. PLOS ONE. 2012;7:e48782.

41. Leitner D, Pires G, Kavanagh T, Kanshin E, Askenazi M, Ueberheide B, et al. Similar brain proteomic signatures in Alzheimer's disease and epilepsy. Acta Neuropathol. 2024 January 30;147:27.

42. Johnson EL, Sullivan KJ, Schneider ALC, Simino J, Mosley TH, Kucharska-Newton A, et al. Association of plasma abeta(42)/abeta(40) ratio and late-onset epilepsy: results from the atherosclerosis risk in communities study. Neurology. 2023 September 26;101:e1319–e1327.

43. Garcia-Cabrero AM, Guerrero-Lopez R, Giraldez BG, Llorens-Martin M, Avila J, Serratosa JM, et al. Hyperexcitability and epileptic seizures in a model of frontotemporal dementia. Neurobiol. Dis. 2013 October;58:200–208.

44. Tai XY, Koepp M, Duncan JS, Fox N, Thompson P, Baxendale S, et al. Hyperphosphorylated tau in patients with refractory epilepsy correlates with cognitive decline: a study of temporal lobe resections. Brain J. Neurol. 2016 September;139:2441–2455.

45. Banote RK, Hakansson S, Zetterberg H, Zelano J. CSF biomarkers in patients with epilepsy in Alzheimer's disease: a nation-wide study. Brain Commun. 2022;4:fcac210.
46. Sherzai D, Losey T, Vega S, Sherzai A. Seizures and dementia in the elderly: nationwide inpatient sample 1999–2008. Epilepsy Behav. 2014 July;36:53–56.
47. Beagle AJ, Darwish SM, Ranasinghe KG, La AL, Karageorgiou E, Vossel KA. Relative incidence of seizures and myoclonus in Alzheimer's disease, dementia with lewy bodies, and frontotemporal dementia. J. Alzheimers Dis. 2017;60:211–223.
48. Mendez MF, Catanzaro P, Doss RC, Arguello R, Frey WH 2nd. Seizures in Alzheimer's disease: clinicopathologic study. J. Geriatr. Psychiatry Neurol. 1994 October–December;7:230–233.
49. Baker J, Libretto T, Henley W, Zeman A. A longitudinal study of epileptic seizures in Alzheimer's disease. Front. Neurol. 2019;10:1266.
50. Amatniek JC, Hauser WA, DelCastillo-Castaneda C, Jacobs DM, Marder K, Bell K, et al. Incidence and predictors of seizures in patients with Alzheimer's disease. Epilepsia. 2006 May;47:867–872.
51. Mahamud Z, Mononen CP, Brigo F, Garcia-Ptacek S, Zelano J. Risk of epilepsy diagnosis after a first unprovoked seizure in dementia. Seizure. 2020 November;82:118–124.
52. Voglein J, Ricard I, Noachtar S, Kukull WA, Dieterich M, Levin J, et al. Seizures in Alzheimer's disease are highly recurrent and associated with a poor disease course. J. Neurol. 2020 October;267:2941–2948.
53. Mendez M, Lim G. Seizures in elderly patients with dementia: epidemiology and management. Drugs Aging. 2003;20:791–803.
54. Jenssen S, Schere D. Treatment and management of epilepsy in the elderly demented patient. Am. J. Alzheimers Dis. Other Demen. 2010 February;25:18–26.
55. Vossel KA, Beagle AJ, Rabinovici GD, Shu H, Lee SE, Naasan G, et al. Seizures and epileptiform activity in the early stages of Alzheimer disease. JAMA Neurol. 2013 September 1;70:1158–1166.
56. Larner AJ. Epileptic seizures in AD patients. Neuromol. Med. 2010 March;12:71–77.
57. Sarkis RA, Dickerson BC, Cole AJ, Chemali ZN. Clinical and neurophysiologic characteristics of unprovoked seizures in patients diagnosed with dementia. J. Neuropsychiatry Clin. Neurosci. 2016 Winter;28:56–61.
58. Horvath A, Szucs A, Hidasi Z, Csukly G, Barcs G, Kamondi A. Prevalence, semiology, and risk factors of epilepsy in Alzheimer's disease: an ambulatory EEG study. J. Alzheimers Dis. 2018;63:1045–1054.
59. Vossel KA, Ranasinghe KG, Beagle AJ, Mizuiri D, Honma SM, Dowling AF, et al. Incidence and impact of subclinical epileptiform activity in Alzheimer's disease. Ann. Neurol. 2016 December;80:858–870.
60. Liedorp M, Stam CJ, van der Flier WM, Pijnenburg YA, Scheltens P. Prevalence and clinical significance of epileptiform EEG discharges in a large memory clinic cohort. Dement. Geriatr. Cogn. Disord. 2010;29:432–437.
61. Larner AJ, Marson AG. Epileptic seizures in Alzheimer's disease: what are the implications of SANAD II? J. Alzheimers Dis. 2022;85:527–529.
62. Liu J, Wang LN, Wu LY, Wang YP. Treatment of epilepsy for people with Alzheimer's disease. Cochrane Database Syst. Rev. 2018 December 20;12:CD011922.
63. Roberson ED, Hope OA, Martin RC, Schmidt D. Geriatric epilepsy: research and clinical directions for the future. Epilepsy Behav. 2011 September;22:103–111.
64. Ferlazzo E, Sueri C, Gasparini S, Aguglia U. Challenges in the pharmacological management of epilepsy and its causes in the elderly. Pharmacol. Res. 2016 April;106:21–26.
65. Cretin B. Pharmacotherapeutic strategies for treating epilepsy in patients with Alzheimer's disease. Expert Opin. Pharmacother. 2018 August;19:1201–1209.
66. Cumbo E, Ligori LD. Levetiracetam, lamotrigine, and phenobarbital in patients with epileptic seizures and Alzheimer's disease. Epilepsy Behav. 2010 April;17:461–466.

67. Hakansson S, Karlander M, Larsson D, Mahamud Z, Garcia-Ptacek S, Zelezniak A, et al. Potential for improved retention rate by personalized antiseizure medication selection: a register-based analysis. Epilepsia. 2021 September;62:2123–2132.
68. Belcastro V, Costa C, Galletti F, Pisani F, Calabresi P, Parnetti L. Levetiracetam mono-therapy in Alzheimer patients with late-onset seizures: a prospective observational study. Eur. J. Neurol. 2007 October;14:1176–1178.
69. Herrmann N, Lanctot KL, Rothenburg LS, Eryavec G. A placebo-controlled trial of val-proate for agitation and aggression in Alzheimer's disease. Dement. Geriatr. Cogn. Disord. 2007;23:116–119.
70. Alsukhni RA, Johnson J, Nashef L. Valproate-induced reversible cognitive decline pre-senting as dementia and associated clinical features: a literature review. Seizure. 2023 October;111:45–50.
71. Sajatovic M, Ramsay E, Nanry K, Thompson T. Lamotrigine therapy in elderly patients with epilepsy, bipolar disorder or dementia. Int. J. Geriatr. Psychiatry. 2007 October;22:945–950.
72. Chin J, Scharfman HE. Shared cognitive and behavioral impairments in epilepsy and Alzhei-mer's disease and potential underlying mechanisms. Epilepsy Behav. 2013 March;26:343–351.
73. Leonard AS, McNamara JO. Does epileptiform activity contribute to cognitive impair-ment in Alzheimer's disease? Neuron. 2007 September 6;55:677–678.
74. Shiozaki K, Kajihara S. Anti-epileptic drugs improved serial 7s scores on the Mini-Mental State Examination in elderly with cognitive impairment and epileptiform discharge on electroencephalography. Psychogeriatrics. 2019;19:38–45.
75. Cretin B, Philippi N, Sellal F, Dibitonto L, Martin-Hunyadi C, Blanc F. Can the syndrome of transient epileptic amnesia be the first feature of Alzheimer's disease? Seizure. 2014 November;23:918–920.
76. Vossel K, Ranasinghe KG, Beagle AJ, La A, Ah Pook K, Castro M, et al. Effect of leve-tiracetam on cognition in patients with Alzheimer disease with and without epileptiform activity: a randomized clinical trial. JAMA Neurol. 2021 November 1;78:1345–1354.
77. Helmstaedter C, Beghi E, Elger CE, Kalviainen R, Malmgren K, May TW, et al. No proof of a causal relationship between antiepileptic drug treatment and incidence of dementia. Comment on: use of antiepileptic drugs and dementia risk—an analysis of Finnish health register and German health insurance data. Epilepsia. 2018 July;59:1303–1306.
78. Taipale H, Gomm W, Broich K, Maier W, Tolppanen AM, Tanskanen A, et al. Use of antiepileptic drugs and dementia risk-an analysis of Finnish Health Register and German Health Insurance Data. J. Am. Geriatr. Soc. 2018 July;66:1123–1129.
79. Breuer LE, Boon P, Bergmans JW, Mess WH, Besseling RM, de Louw A, et al. Cognitive deterioration in adult epilepsy: does accelerated cognitive ageing exist? Neurosci. Biobehav. Rev. 2016 May;64:1–11.
80. Breuer LEM, Grevers E, Boon P, Bernas A, Bergmans JWM, Besseling RMH, et al. Cognitive deterioration in adult epilepsy: clinical characteristics of "accelerated cognitive ageing." Acta Neurol. Scand. 2017 July;136:47–53.
81. McAreavey MJ, Ballinger BR, Fenton GW. Epileptic seizures in elderly patients with dementia. Epilepsia. 1992 July–August;33:657–660.
82. Bjellvi J, Idegard A, Zelano J. Risk factors for status epilepticus after brain disorders in adults: a multi-cohort national register study. Epilepsy Behav. 2024 July;156:109840.
83. Puteikis K, Mameniskiene R. Mortality among people with epilepsy: a retrospective nationwide analysis from 2016 to 2019. Int. J. Environ. Res. Public Health. 2021 October 7;18:10512.
84. Sveinsson O, Andersson T, Carlsson S, Tomson T. Type, etiology, and duration of epi-lepsy as risk factors for SUDEP: further analyses of a population-based case-control study. Neurology. 2023 November 27;101:e2257–e2265.
85. Vossel KA, Beagle AJ, Rabinovici GD, Shu H, Lee SE, et al. Seizures and epilepti-form activity in the early stages of Alzheimer disease. JAMA Neurol. 2013 September 1;70:1158–1166.

Epilepsy in Brain Tumors

7

7.1 RISK OF EPILEPSY

Brain tumors account for approximately 5%–10% of all epilepsy, and overall, 50% of patients with primary brain tumors or metastases will have seizures during the course of their disease.[1] Patients are seen in neuro-oncology, neurology, oncology, neurosurgery, and internal medicine, which has given rise to an interesting literature with different perspectives. For instance, recent advances in neurosurgery, neuropathology, and oncology have provided complementary insights into tumor-related epileptogenesis. Different tumors have different risks of epilepsy (Figure 7.1), and the risk can sometimes, but not always, be reduced with tumor treatment.

Brain tumors of very low grade can be the cause of medically refractory epilepsy and removed in epilepsy surgery, but this chapter will mainly discuss brain tumors often encountered in everyday health care and general neurology: gliomas, meningiomas, and metastases.

7.1.1 Gliomas

Gliomas and glioblastoma are primary brain tumors. The risk of epilepsy in gliomas is highly related to tumor grade, with lower-grade tumors being more common in patients where the tumor is detected because of new-onset seizures.[2] In gliomas grade II (diffuse oligodentroglioma and astrocytoma) with isocitrate dehydrogenase (IDH)-mutation, at least two thirds of patients will have seizures.[3–6] In higher-grade gliomas, the risk is slightly lower, and in grade IV tumors—glioblastomas—only one third of patients have seizures as their presenting symtom.[1,6]

Importantly, the risks are dynamic and dependent on when the tumor is detected. For instance, a substantial proportion of glioblastoma patients will develop seizures during the course of the disease, but many have seizures just in the final months. In low-grade gliomas, seizures are often the presenting symptom and because the tumors occur frequently in young adults, epilepsy can be a major contributor to morbidity throughout the disease course.

DOI: 10.1201/9781003501404-7

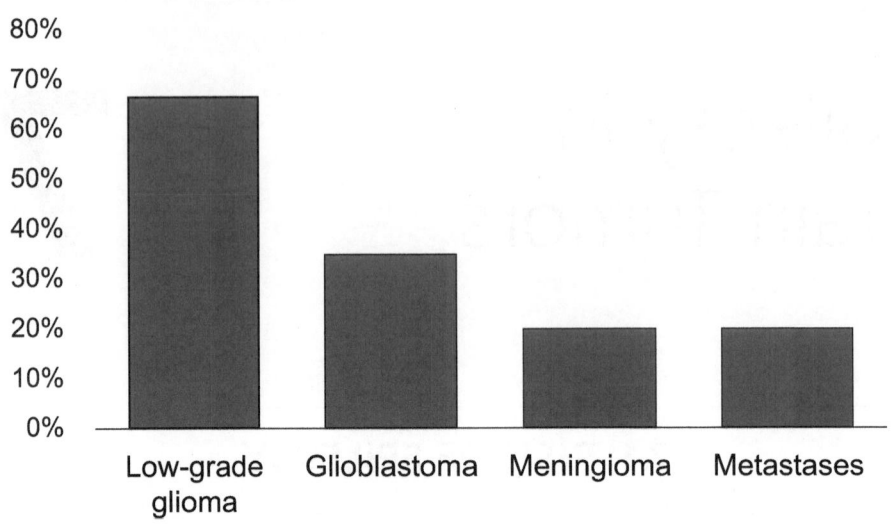

FIGURE 7.1   Estimated proportion of patients with epilepsy in different tumor types.

7.1.2 Meningiomas

Meningiomas are common primary CNS tumors. The risk of epilepsy is difficult to assess; there are many large case series from surgical centers describing that about 30%–50% of treated patients had seizures before their surgery,[1] but how many in the catchment area of that surgical center that were never referred is rarely known. Overall, around 20% of all patients with meningiomas are estimated to have seizures.[7–9] Seizures are more common prior to surgery but may continue after in a few patients.

7.1.3 Metastases

Brain metastases are common, but an unresearched field. Perhaps as many as one fifth of all cancers result in brain metastases, which in turn cause a large proportion of all tumor-related epilepsy. In patients with brain metastases, about 10%–35% will have seizures.[1,4,10,11] Malignant melanoma seems to be a tumor particularly prone to cause epilepsy.[11]

7.1.4 Other Tumors

There are several rarer brain tumors that can cause epilepsy. Dysembryoplastic neu-roepithelial tumors, DNET, are low-grade tumors causing epilepsy in most patients. Gangliogliomas are another low-grade tumor that cause seizures in 80% of treated cases.[1] The term low-grade epilepsy-associated neuroepithelial tumors (LEAT) designates other difficult-to-classify but most often benign glioneuronal or neuronal tumors found in work-up of pharmacoresistant epilepsy.[6]

In tumor syndromes, the risk varies but is higher than in the general population. In a case series of adults with neurofibromatosis (NF) type I, the life prevalence of epilepsy (median age of the 11 patients was 33) was 11% and the point prevalence 7%. Somewhat less than half of the cases did not seem to be caused by an intracranial tumor, and in 18% onset of epilepsy preceded the diagnosis of NF1, suggesting epileptogenic mechanisms other than structural expansivity.[12] Similarly, epilepsy is common in tuberous sclerosis, affecting about 90%.[13]

7.2 EPILEPTOGENESIS

The epileptogenesis of brain tumors have been increasingly understood in the last years, through advances in imaging, genetics, and neuropathology. The ways brain tumors can cause epilepsy include mass effect disrupting adjacent cortical function, edema favoring an excitotoxic environment, glial changes affecting the microenvironment, glutamate receptor agonists being secreted by tumor cells, and direct contacts with neurons in gliomaneuronal synapses (Figure 7.2). The key brain area seems to be the immediate vicinity of the tumor, sometimes interacting with the tumor tissue itself.[1] Elucidating which mechanisms are at work in which patients harbors great potential for future personalized medicine.

7.2.1 Gliomas

Gliomas are believed to cause seizures by most of the mechanisms previously listed, including mass effect, edema, glial changes, excitotoxic substances, and direct effects on neurons including tumor-neuronal contacts.

Mass effect disrupts cortical function by pressing on brain tissue, presumably restricting perfusion and causing neuronal dysfunction. It can also cause gliosis, with particularly astrocytes reacting to the microenvironment changes with gliosis—which

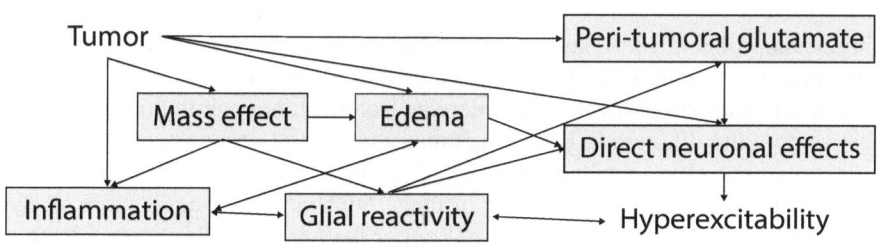

FIGURE 7.2   Examples of epileptogenic mechanisms in tumor-related epilepsy.

can in itself favor an excitotoxic environment (discussed later). Edema is closely related to mass effect and related to both growth size and type of the glioma. Edema is usually present in the peritumeral area but can extend substantially. It is an independent risk factor for seizures in low-grade gliomas and believed to promote epileptogenesis.[5] The microcellular environment harbors a lot of glutamate and seems to promote a shift in both neuronal and glial function. Some of this effect may be mediated through inflammatory cascades; the peritumeral area is full of activated astrocytes, microglia, and macrophages as well as interleukins like IL-1beta and IL-6 promoting neuronal hyperexcitability.[1] The anatomical extension of the tumor is also likely to be important, with PET studies showing that metabolic volume and extension into the temporal lobe are associated with epilepsy.[14] Smaller tumor volume is sometimes associated with seizures, but the extent to which this reflects actual differences in tumor biology in smaller tumors or simply that seizures have led to diagnosis is difficult to disentangle.[6]

Gliomas also affect astrocytes, microglia, and neurons directly. The environment around a tumor is hyperexcitable.[6] Some glioma cells actively secrete glutamate or glutamate receptor agonists. Meanwhile, astrocytes close to tumors are reactive and less effective in removing glutamate from the extracellular space.[6] Taken together, this may shift the excitatory/inhibitory balance or increase the "glutamatergic tone."[1] The role of microglia is unclear. They are activated peritumorally, but whether this is reactive or not is unknown, and in mouse models ablation of microglia aggravates seizures.[15] Neurons themselves feature relatively more excitatory synapses in the vicinity of gliomas. Finally, tumor cells can directly contact neurons in so-called neurogliomal synapses, which are excitatory through AMPA-glutamate receptors.[1] These connections and tumor growth may be stimulated by neurotrophic factors released by neuronal activity, so one can speculate that seizures may be detrimental for tumor prognosis. This is so far a theory, but one that has given rise to some interesting trial ideas (discussed later).

The genetics of gliomas also influence epileptogenesis.[2] IDH mutation increases the risk of seizures,[5] perhaps by increasing expulsion of a glutamate agonist from tumor cells.[1] Gliomas with IDH mutations also seem more likely to influence neighboring neurons and promote a hyperexcitable state. Conversely, IDH wildtype glioblastoma have relatively low risk of seizures at diagnosis. The risk rises during the disease course, presumably as other mechanisms including mass effect and gliosis become more important.[16]

7.2.2 Meningiomas

Meningiomas probably cause seizures by some mechanisms also used by gliomas—namely mass effect, edema, and glial reactivity.[17] Being extra-axial tumors, most meningiomas have less access to the cortical microenvironment, but meningiomas with more infiltrative growth—like grade II meningiomas and grade I secretory meningiomas (a rare type)—seem to have much higher risk of seizures.[17] There are also meningioma-specific genetics being investigated; for instance NF2 mutation seems more likely to promote epilepsy, perhaps through atypical tumor features including more edema and brain invasion.[17] Surgery is successful in stopping seizures in most cases, but some patients with meningioma-induced seizures continue to have epilepsy after removal, demonstrating that some epileptogenic changes could be permanent and not merely reflect mass effect or edema.

7.2.3 Other Tumors

For brain metastases, some cancers like melanoma and small cell lung cancer seem more likely to cause seizures than others.[11] Some tumors like DNET and ganglioglioma are extremely slow growing so mass effect is less likely to play a major role in epileptogenesis. Many of these tumors have altered cortical morphology in their immediate surroundings resembling dysplasias, but there is also inflammation.[6,18] In tuberous sclerosis, hyperactivation of the mTOR pathway is believed to drive both epileptogenesis and tumor growth.[6,13]

7.3 RISK FACTORS

Clinical risk factors for tumor-related epilepsy include young age but otherwise vary between different tumor types (Table 7.1).

7.3.1 Gliomas

Young age, low-grade tumor, IDH mutation, and edema are the strongest risk factors for epilepsy in gliomas. The risk of seizures varies through the disease course. In low-grade gliomas, the risk of seizures is reduced by tumor treatment. All modalities (radiotherapy, surgery, and chemotherapy) reduce the risk of seizures, but estimating seizure risk in individual patients after different treatments is not yet possible. An important clinical point is that recurrence of seizures after tumor treatment can indicate tumor relapse.

Patients with IDH wildtype glioblastoma have a relatively low risk of seizures at presentation (33%), but this rises throughout the disease course to over 50%. Risk factors for brain tumor–related epilepsy are younger age and contrast enhancement. Factors that are more difficult to interpret but also related to epilepsy are low tumor volume and longer time to diagnosis from symptom onset, but these may reflect when the tumor was detected rather than intrinsic tumor factors. Risk factors for poor seizure control throughout the disease course are previously uncontrolled seizures, tonic-clonic seizures, and limited surgical resection.[16]

7.3.2 Meningiomas

High-grade meningiomas, infiltrative growth, large volume, edema, and age are associated with seizures in meningioma, and in a multivariable analysis of these, younger age,

TABLE 7.1   Some Reported Risk Factors for Epilepsy in Different Tumors

GLIOMAS	MENINGIOMAS	METASTASES
Young age	Young age	Primary tumor type
Low-grade	Edema	Location
IDH mutation	Location	Whole brain radiation
Edema	Size	Radiotherapy

edema, and location of the meningioma were associated with preoperative seizures.[8,19] Sex is sometimes discussed as a risk factor, with males more often having seizures despite females more often having meningiomas.[9,17] Preoperative seizures are a risk factor for postoperative seizures, but development of new-onset epilepsy after meningioma surgery seems relatively rare.[8,9,17,19] If seizures are uncontrolled before surgery, the risk is increased about two- to three-fold that they will continue after.[17]

7.3.3 Metastases

The risk of seizures differs between metastases from different cancers, suggesting that different tumors induce different epileptogenic processes. Metastases from malignant melanoma seem particularly prone to cause epilepsy.[11] Other risk factors for seizures in patients with brain metastases are radiotherapy, whole brain radiation, and tumors in particular locations. Whole brain radiation is perhaps a marker of total tumor load.

7.4 MANAGEMENT

7.4.1 Clinical Presentation

Tumor-related seizures are focal, and if motor they affect the contralateral side.[1] Seizures can evolve rapidly into bilateral tonic-clonic seizures, and the focal onset may be clinically imperceptible. The proportions of different seizure types vary between studies. In glioblastoma, one large case series found that at presentation 55% had focal motor seizures without impaired awareness, 17% had focal seizures with impaired awareness, and 29% had bilateral tonic-clonic seizures.[16] For low-grade gliomas, a large meta-analysis showed that 42% of seizures were focal, 37% were tonic-clonic, and 21% were other (presumably focal non-motor) seizures.[3] For meningiomas, the proportion of seizures are relatively similar. Motor seizures were the most common in one series, accounting for nearly 80%, and somatosensory seizures were the most common non-motor seizure type.[8]

7.4.1.1 Status Epilepticus

Status epilepticus was until recently not considered very common in brain tumor–related epilepsy.[1] The kind of status epilepticus can range from convulsive to non-convulsive, and focal motor status (epilepsia partialis continua) is sometimes encountered in patients with brain tumors. One interesting recent cohort study showed that although status epilepticus may perhaps be seldomly encountered among patients with brain tumors, it is not a rare status epilepticus etiology from a neurological care perspective. The authors found status epilepticus in 182 patients with brain tumors (85 gliomas, 77 metastases, and 20 other brain tumors) among a total of 961 status epilepticus episodes in over 800 patients,[20] so brain tumors accounted for almost 20% of status epilepticus episodes. In 33 patients, the brain tumor was diagnosed because status epilepticus was the presenting symptom. Compared to non-neoplastic cases of status epilepticus, patients with brain tumors had less impairment of consciousness and convulsive status epilepticus was less common.

7.4.2 Estimating Recurrence Risk after a First Seizure

Contrary to the case for the other brain conditions discussed in the book, in which epilepsy arises as a consequence of a previous brain disorder, diagnosis of a brain tumor tends to overshadow epilepsy aspects. The recurrence risk is probably high, at least in gliomas. This is reflected in most consensus documents, according to which a first seizure seems to be considered as epilepsy in most patients with brain tumors.[1]

Acute symptomatic seizures can occur in brain tumors, but there is very little robust evidence to guide management. What constitutes an acute symptomatic seizure or not in brain tumor–related epilepsy is a matter of clinical judgment. Tumor bleeds or other temporary deterioration may perhaps cause acute symptomatic seizures that do not indicate epilepsy (an enduring predisposition for seizures). In most cases, considering a first seizure epilepsy seems to be a pragmatic and reasonable approach. Actual recurrence risks are hard to determine, since most studies do not provide detailed epilepsy follow-up. A recent prospective study of first seizures found tumors to confer the highest recurrence risk among remote etiologies, over the ILAE 60% threshold required for an epilepsy diagnosis.[21] Since recurrence risks probably differ between tumor types,[22] this is a relatively crude estimate.

7.4.3 Risks of Seizure Recurrence in Different Tumors

Studies describing first seizure recurrence risks for specific tumors are rare. Just like for prevalence, some results can be inferred from surgically treated series, but these could be biased in that patients with more seizures could be accepted for surgery more often. One such study reported that 38% of patients with seizures before resection of meningiomas had more than one preoperative seizure.[23] The recurrence risk after a first postoperative seizure after meningioma surgery is not well characterized.[24] In gliomas, seizure risks are related to tumor histology and progression.[25-27] In surgically treated patients with seizures in glioma, more than one preoperative seizure has been reported in >60%,[28,29] suggesting that most patients have epilepsy. A particularly important aspect of management of first seizures in gliomas is that seizures are a typical symptom at onset for low-grade tumors. If seizures develop later in the disease course, it could be an indication of tumor progression warranting radiology.[25]

CASE 7.1 First Seizure

A 65-year-old male presents with a first seizure and the work-up reveals glioblastoma. He is started on levetiracetam and considered non-operable. Instead, he receives chemotherapy. His wife asks if the ASM is really necessary since he has only had one seizure.

> *Comment: There is no good data on seizure recurrence risks in brain tumors, but the expert consensus is that a single seizure in the presence of a glioma/glioblastoma/metastasis motivates treatment in most cases.*

The risk of seizure recurrence after a first seizure in brain metastases is largely unknown, and clinical practice typically derives from experience with primary brain tumors. It is reasonable to assume a high recurrence risk,[1] and the advanced cancer indicated by presence of a brain metastasis typically draws attention from semantics of whether epilepsy is present.

These recurrence risks mean that in both primary tumors and metastases, most experts currently find it reasonable to recommend ASM treatment after a first seizure. Guidelines do not recommend ASM therapy before the first seizure in brain tumors, although in practice this is sometimes administered (discussed later).

7.4.4 Treatment of Epilepsy

There is no strong evidence to suggest that a particular ASM is better than any other with regards to suppressing seizures in brain tumor patients.[1] Instead, ASMs are selected—as in all other epilepsies—with patient and seizure/epilepsy factors in mind. Since seizures in brain tumor–related epilepsies are focal, ASMs registered for focal epilepsy are reasonable options.

It is important to weigh pros and cons of ASM therapy individually. Patients with brain tumors can find that seizures reduce quality of life by causing anxiety and concern, memory impairment, and driving inability and by requiring daily medications. Conversely, ASM side effects also impact quality of life if cognitive dysfunction and fatigue become too prominent.[7]

In most guidelines or expert opinions, prophylactic ASM treatment in patients with brain tumors who have not had a seizure is not recommended.[1,9] There are a few randomized trials on the matter in gliomas. The reason for not recommending primary prophylaxis is that ASMs have side effects and that many patients will need to be unnecessarily treated to prevent a first seizure. Despite this, practice varies across regions. Within Europe, survey responses indicate that prophylaxis habits vary between countries.[4] It is also important to note that many studies regarding ASM treatment involved patients using older-generation ASMs with substantial side effects. It is possible that newer ASMs have fewer cognitive side effects and that at some point precision medicine or other prediction tools will allow identification of patients with a particularly high risk of seizures in which prophylaxis may be motivated.

Multidisciplinary collaboration is required in most patients with brain tumor–related epilepsy. In addition to control of epilepsy, tumor treatment, comorbidities, and psychosocial factors like driving need to be addressed in most patients. An important aspect concerns radiological surveillance, which must be tailored according to the underlying tumor type and treatment received.

In the final stages of brain tumor care, IV access may not be available and oral administration of tablets impossible because of somnolence. Clonazepam and midazolam are some alternatives mentioned in reviews as options that can be administered in droplets, intranasally or buccally.[10]

7.4.4.1 Status Epilepticus

Status epilepticus is managed according to local guidelines. A recent case series of over 182 patients described that levetiracetam was the most commonly used ASM following bensodiazepines.[20] Other options utilized were valproate and lacosamide. The study was retrospective but revealed no differences in efficacy between these ASMs. The effect of ASMs on seizure cessation was slightly higher in patients with brain tumors than in status epilepticus in general, but individual prediction is difficult. The study also supports the popularity of newer ASMs like levetiracetam and perhaps lacosamide in status epilepticus treatment of patients with brain tumors, since these have a more favorable pharmacological profile regarding drug–drug interactions than older options like phenytoin.

7.4.4.2 Gliomas

When selecting an ASM for patients with glioma one must take patient demographics, comorbidities, seizure severity, and tumor characteristics into account. For instance, very sparse seizures may allow titration of lamotrigine or other ASMs that take a while to reach therapeutic doses, whereas frequent seizures may require an ASM that can reach a therapeutic dose more rapidly. It is often advisable to avoid drugs with too many drug–drug interactions, like hepatic enzyme inducers (carbamazepine, phenytoin, etc.).[2] Valproic acid is often reported as a treatment in older glioma series but has drawbacks with high protein binding, potential for drug interaction, and potentially severe side effects including encephalopathy. It is also contraindicated in pregnancy and in women of childbearing age. Current reviews favor levetiracetam or lacosamide before valproate, which is perhaps best reserved for cases needing add-on treatment for seizure control.[1] The most commonly used ASM currently seems to be levetiracetam,[16] but lacosamide, lamotrigine, valproic acid, clobazam, topiramate, and zonisamide are also mentioned in reviews of treatment options.[1,2] Individualized ASM selection, just like in any epilepsy, seems to be the best approach currently.

In studies evaluating efficacy (absence of treatment failure), levetiracetam usually performs well. The drug is favored in brain tumor patients because of its lack of drug–drug interactions and was the most common choice in a survey of European neuro-oncology centers, regardless of whether seizures were focal or bilateral tonic-clonic.[4] Mood and other psychiatric side effects are important to monitor for.[1] In case of an ineffective first monotherapy, an alternative monotherapy or combination therapy can be attempted just like for other epilepsies. European neuro-oncologists answered in a survey that they considered valproate and lacosamide equivalent first monotherapy options to levetiracetam, but of course surveys are not to be confused with actual evidence.[4]

If seizure control is considered of importance for quality of life and a first monotherapy fails, add-on therapy can be a reasonable second regime. Some experts advocate a policy of rational polytherapy, selecting add-on treatment with an alternative mechanism of action than the baseline therapy, which may also have the benefit of reducing side effects. Levetiracetam with valproate has been reported as an effective combination, as has phenytoin and levetiracetam, but the latter combination has significant drawbacks because of enzyme induction.[1] Lacosamide or perampanel have also reported as suitable add-on therapies,[1,30] but comparative studies between most polytherapies are missing. Some 15% of glioblastoma and 40% of lower-grade gliomas are medically refractory, and patients continue to have seizures despite having tried two ASMs.[1]

With an underlying neoplastic disease, the question often arises if changes in epilepsy symptoms reflect tumor progression. The issue is exquisitely difficult to study systematically, and clinical judgment is the best guide. Some systematic follow-ups of larger patient series express the opinion that seizures rarely present during stable tumor disease.[25] In extension, this could translate to a clinical approach in which seizure recurrence after long seizure freedom, new semiology, or new development of seizure clusters probably should warrant neuroradiology to look for tumor progression.

ASMs AS TUMOR DRUGS?

There is a discussion and some studies investigating whether ASMs themselves can have an impact on tumor treatment or progression.[2,31] Valproic acid has been speculated to potentiate chemotherapy, fell out of favor, but is now again investigated in such studies with varying results. Similarly, perampanel is currently being considered as an anti-tumoral agent due to the expression of AMPA receptors by glioma cells and the possibility of interference with growth-stimulating signaling, potentially involving glioma-neuronal synapses. So far, meta-analyses of existing studies have not shown any clear benefit on survival.[10] Recent larger studies do not support increased survival in brain tumor patients with adjunctive ASMs, in fact some studies even report worse survival for patients on some ASMs,[32] but it is an evolving field.

7.4.4.3 Meningiomas

ASM treatment of meningioma-related seizures follows the same principles as those in glioma. Particularly levetiracetam is mentioned as a common monotherapy treatment option, but any ASM is possible to use with the normal considerations of patient characteristics taken into account.[9,17] In one large series, perampanel was prescribed as first add-on treatment,[8] but evidence of differential efficacy of different combinations is not available and tradition probably varies between countries. Older drugs like valproate and phenobarbital are still mentioned in the literature, but drug–drug interaction and side effects have hopefully reduced the appeal of these drugs in the future in favor of newer ASMs.

7.4.4.4 Metastases

Brain metastases are difficult to investigate in isolation, and most treatment guidelines derive from conclusions based on gliomas or meningiomas. There may be differences between different primary tumors, with malignant melanoma being among those with a particularly high seizure risk, but there is no high-level evidence to guide ASM selection.[1]

7.4.4.5 Side Effects

Side effects can be particularly problematic in brain tumor patients. Clinical judgment is required to correctly weigh the drawbacks of memory impairment and tiredness against the benefits of seizure freedom. Sometimes total seizure freedom is not achievable with acceptable quality of life. Shared decision-making is paramount.

7.4.5 Withdrawal

7.4.5.1 Gliomas

Just like add-on therapy may be required if seizures continue, ASMs can sometimes be reduced after tumor treatment. It is important to remember that individual prediction of seizure recurrence risks is not possible and that tapering and the consequences of seizure relapse need to be discussed with the patient carefully, just like in all epilepsy. Seizures as well as side effects have negative effects on quality of life, and a consensus paper mentions that two years of seizure freedom might be a reasonable balance between avoiding too early tapering and too long exposure to ASM side effects.[7] A survey of European neuro-oncology centers showed that 47% of respondents would consider reducing the dose if patients with a low-grade glioma were seizure free after tumor treatment, but only 30% in high-grade glioma.[4] Careful consideration before withdrawal is probably best also in low-grade tumors—the risk of seizure recurrence varies considerably in the literature. Patients with maximal safe resection have been suggested as a group in which ASM withdrawal can be considered. If seizures do recur, especially after a longer latency, it is important to remember that this might indicate tumor recurrence or progression.[7]

CASE 7.2 Withdrawal

A 45-year-old man has focal motor impaired awareness seizures and the work-up reveals a low-grade glioma. He is started on levetiracetam, which reduces the semiology, and undergoes surgery with gross total resection that goes well. He and his family ask about stopping the antiseizure medication now that the tumor has been removed. He has had one small seizure after the surgery.

Comment: Although there is insufficient evidence, most expert opinions advise that a period of seizure freedom is appropriate before tapering ASMs. Two to five years is generally considered suitable. This patient does not seem seizure free—which argues strongly against stopping the treatment. Understanding and addressing concerns that can be the reason for the patient's wish to stop the ASM is important—are there side effects or misconceptions either about the effect of the ASM or the chronicity of the brain tumor condition? If there are side effects, another ASM may be a suitable course of action. Clinical judgment and shared decision-making are essential in balancing side effects against seizure risks to minimize the impact on quality of life.

7.4.5.2 Meningiomas

A difficult question is whether ASMs can be tapered after meningioma surgery in patients with preoperative seizures. Estimates suggest that most patients will become seizure free after surgery, but a substantial proportion will continue to have seizures and data are simply not available for more individualized prediction.[17] Most experts recommend maintaining ASM therapy for at least one to two years after surgery.[9] Nonetheless, meningioma was the tumor type in which most European doctors at neuro-oncology centers would consider tapering out of all brain tumors.[4] It is important to note the different risks in different meningioma grades; experts have suggested that ASM withdrawal can be considered in grade I meningiomas with maximal resection but not in higher-grade meningiomas if the patient has ever had a seizure.[7] As in all other epilepsy, a period of seizure freedom is probably advisable and shared decision-making before ASMs are reduced. It is important that patients understand the risks of tapering—including implications for driving and seizure-related risks like falls.

7.4.5.3 Metastases

With regards to the tapering of ASMs after tumor treatment, a survey suggests that metastases are the tumor type for which the fewest doctors working in neuro-oncology would consider reducing ASMs.[4]

7.4.6 Non-ASM Treatment

Most treatment besides ASMs relates to the tumor disease itself, but radiotherapy, surgery, and chemotherapy are beyond the scope of this book. All of these therapies can reduce seizures. Similarly, corticosteroids for the edema around a tumor can sometimes improve seizure control but are rarely used alone without ASMs. The impact of different non-medical treatments on seizures and the clinical considerations that follow are briefly discussed next.

7.4.6.1 Surgery

Gliomas can be treated with surgery, radiotherapy, and/or chemotherapy. Gross total resection seems to result in superior seizure outcomes in most brain tumor types, and it seems even better if the border around the tumor has also been removed.[1,3] In meningiomas, surgical resection results in seizure freedom in about 70% (53%–90%), so the prognosis is relatively good but not without risk of postoperative seizures.[9,17,19] The decision to offer surgery is individualized, and seizures are most often considered an indication only if uncontrolled by medical therapy.[9] Some authors discuss that an epilepsy-surgery approach to meningioma removal could be suitable in certain select cases, if there are refractory seizures and extensive gliosis, particularly in the temporal lobe.[17]

7.4.6.2 Radiotherapy

Radiotherapy has been reported to improve seizures in both low- and high-grade gliomas, with responder rates (at least 50% seizure reduction) reported in up to 77% in certain series and seizure freedom in 38%.[1]

7.4.6.3 Chemotherapy and Other Drugs

Chemotherapy including temozolomide improves seizures in some patients, and seizure freedom has been reported in up to 50% of some treated series.[1] The mTOR inhibitor everolimus is used in tuberous sclerosis to treat both tumors and epilepsy. Radiological monitoring is important, and current practice is to monitor for giant cell astrocytoma development well into adulthood.

7.5 PROGNOSIS

7.5.1 Seizures

Most brain-tumor related epilepsy can be controlled with ASMs, at least initially (Table 7.2). In low-grade gliomas, a meta-analysis found factors associated with postoperative freedom to be focal seizures as opposed to bilateral tonic-clonic ones and extent of resection. Other adjuvant therapy did not impact the outcome, but gross total

TABLE 7.2   Risk Factors of Pharmacoresistance

Tumor grade and type
Gross total resection
Bilateral tonic-clonic seizures
Status epilepticus

resection increased the likelihood of seizure freedom at least four times.[3] The findings give some suggestion to important factors, but the individual decisions about appropriateness for and timing of neurosurgery make firm conclusions difficult. Some estimates indicate that 50% of all glioma patients continue to have seizures despite monotherapy,[1] but the figure is probably higher for low-grade gliomas and lower for glioblastoma. In the latter, seizure control is usually achieved with monotherapy for 85% early in the disease course but worsens later. At the end-of-life phase approximately half of patients with glioblastoma have epilepsy, and 30%–40% of these have seizures despite therapy.[7,16] In meningiomas, most patients will be seizure free after surgery.

7.5.2 Quality of Life

With improved treatment of brain tumors, particularly of childhood and low-grade glioma forms, increasing numbers of brain tumor survivors have to deal with consequences of their disease, including seizures. A qualitative study inventorying self-management aspects in patients with low-grade glioma found that seizures had a significant impact on quality of life, more specifically as a barrier to independence.[33] Driving and swimming were activities that participants mentioned missing, and memory problems caused significant problems for some. Seizures themselves were also mentioned, specifically concern about them in social circumstances. Tiredness and feeling mentally drained were other important barriers. This fits well with studies on the low-grade glioma population in general, in which tiredness and cognitive symptoms are important determinants of quality of life.[34] Such symptoms are also common side effects of antiseizure medications.

For clinicians, the aforementioned study and others like it hold important lessons. Unnecessary ASM drug load should be avoided to minimize side effects like tiredness and memory decline. At the same time, seizures and concern for seizures are also important. Clearly, the patient knows best how to weigh the relative pros and cons of ASM treatment versus seizure risk. A personalized approach with individualized goals is most often beneficial (Table 7.3).

7.5.3 Survival

In low-grade glioma, the presence of seizures at onset is associated with longer survival, but there is less data on the impact of epilepsy that ensued during the course of the disease.[35] The issue is difficult to study, since seizures are such a common presenting

TABLE 7.3   Clinical Take-Home Messages

- 50% of patients with primary brain tumors or metastases will have seizures during the course of their disease.
- Seizures are often a presenting symptom. Risks of further seizures are high, and most experts advocate ASM therapy after a first seizure.
- Tumor treatment like surgery and chemotherapy can often improve seizure control, but particularly in progressive tumor types like gliomas, higher-grade meningiomas, and metastases, recurrence risks are high.
- Most experts recommend at least a few years of seizure freedom before reduction of ASMs is considered. Reduction of doses may be preferable to complete withdrawal. Shared decision-making is essential, so that the patient understands the risks of seizure recurrence.
- Several ASMs are used for treatment of tumor-related epilepsy; levetiracetam seems common at the moment.
- Seizure recurrence after tumor treatment may indicate tumor relapse or progression, and neuroimaging is often indicated.

symptom. One series suggested that absence of seizure freedom in the early stages of low-grade glioma could be linked to a worse prognosis.[35] Similarly, seizures as a presenting symptom is a favorable prognostic marker in glioblastoma.[16]

REFERENCES

1. Newton HB, Wojkowski J. Antiepileptic strategies for patients with primary and metastatic brain tumors. Curr. Treat. Options Oncol. 2024 March;25:389–403.
2. Avila EK, Tobochnik S, Inati SK, Koekkoek JAF, McKhann GM, Riviello JJ, et al. Brain tumor-related epilepsy management: a Society for Neuro-oncology (SNO) consensus review on current management. Neurol. Oncol. 2024 January 5;26:7–24.
3. Nandoliya KR, Thirunavu V, Ellis E, Dixit K, Tate MC, Drumm MR, et al. Pre-operative predictors of post-operative seizure control in low-grade glioma: a systematic review and meta-analysis. Neurosurg. Rev. 2024 February 27;47:94.
4. van der Meer PB, Dirven L, van den Bent MJ, Preusser M, Taphoorn MJB, Ruda R, et al. Prescription preferences of antiepileptic drugs in brain tumor patients: an international survey among EANO members. Neurooncol. Pract. 2022 April;9:105–113.
5. Tang T, Wang Y, Dai Y, Liu Q, Fan X, Cheng Y, et al. IDH1 mutation predicts seizure occurrence and prognosis in lower-grade glioma adults. Pathol. Res. Pract. 2024 February;254:155165.
6. Ruda R, Bruno F, Pellerino A. Epilepsy in gliomas: recent insights into risk factors and molecular pathways. Curr. Opin. Neurol. 2023 December 1;36:557–563.
7. Peters KB, Templer J, Gerstner ER, Wychowski T, Storstein AM, Dixit K, et al. Discontinuation of antiseizure medications in patients with brain tumors. Neurology. 2024 February 27;102:e209163.
8. Pauletto G, Nilo A, Pez S, Zonta ME, Bagatto D, Isola M, et al. Meningioma related epilepsy: a happy ending? J. Pers. Med. 2023 July 11;13:1124.

9. Peart R, Melnick K, Cibula J, Walbert T, Gerstner ER, Rahman M, et al. Clinical management of seizures in patients with meningiomas: efficacy of surgical resection for seizure control and patient-tailored postoperative anti-epileptic drug management. Neurooncol. Adv. 2023 May;5:i58–i66.

10. van der Meer PB, Taphoorn MJB, Koekkoek JAF. Management of epilepsy in brain tumor patients. Curr. Opin. Oncol. 2022 November 1;34:685–690.

11. Lamba N, Catalano PJ, Cagney DN, Haas-Kogan DA, Bubrick EJ, Wen PY, et al. Seizures among patients with brain metastases: a population- and institutional-level analysis. Neurology. 2021 February 22;96:e1237–e1250.

12. Hebert J, De Santis RJ, Daniyal L, Mannan S, Ng E, Thain E, et al. Epilepsy in neurofibromatosis type 1: prevalence, phenotype, and genotype in adults. Epilepsy Res. 2024 March 2;202:107336.

13. Vitale G, Terrone G, Vitale S, Vitulli F, Aiello S, Bravaccio C, et al. The evolving landscape of therapeutics for epilepsy in tuberous sclerosis complex. Biomedicines. 2023 December 7;11:3241.

14. Bono BC, Ninatti G, Riva M, Raspagliesi L, Barbieri EM, Navarria P, et al. The role of preoperative [11C]methionine PET in defining tumor-related epilepsy and predicting short-term postoperative seizure control in temporal lobe low-grade gliomas. Neurosurg. Focus. 2024 February;56:E6.

15. Gibbs-Shelton S, Benderoth J, Gaykema RP, Straub J, Okojie KA, Uweru JO, et al. Microglia play beneficial roles in multiple experimental seizure models. Glia. 2023 July;71:1699–1714.

16. Pallud J, Roux A, Moiraghi A, Aboubakr O, Elia A, Guinard E, et al. Characteristics and prognosis of tumor-related epilepsy during tumor evolution in patients with IDH wild-type glioblastoma. Neurology. 2024 January 9;102:e207902.

17. Dincer A, Jalal MI, Gupte TP, Vetsa S, Vasandani S, Yalcin K, et al. The clinical and genomic features of seizures in meningiomas. Neurooncol. Adv. 2023 May;5:i49–i57.

18. Liu Q, Cai L, Sun Y, Wang Y, Yu H, Liu C, et al. Epilepsy outcome and pathology analysis for ganglioglioma: a series of 51 pediatric patients. Pediatr. Neurol. 2023 December;149:127–133.

19. Bogdanovic I, Ristic A, Ilic R, Bascarevic V, Bukumiric Z, Miljkovic A, et al. Factors associated with preoperative and early and late postoperative seizures in patients with supratentorial meningiomas. Epileptic. Disord. 2023 April;25:244–254.

20. Tziakouri A, Hottinger AF, Novy J, Rossetti AO. Status epilepticus management in patients with brain tumors: a cohort study. Seizure. 2024 June 6;120:1–4.

21. Lawn N, Chan J, Lee J, Dunne J. Is the first seizure epilepsy —and when? Epilepsia. 2015 September;56:1425–1431.

22. van Breemen MS, Wilms EB, Vecht CJ. Epilepsy in patients with brain tumours: epidemiology, mechanisms, and management. Lancet Neurol. 2007 May;6:421–430.

23. Chaichana KL, Pendleton C, Zaidi H, Olivi A, Weingart JD, Gallia GL, et al. Seizure control for patients undergoing meningioma surgery. World Neurosurg. 2013 March–April;79:515–524.

24. Xue H, Sveinsson O, Tomson T, Mathiesen T. Intracranial meningiomas and seizures: a review of the literature. Acta Neurochir (Wien). 2015 September;157:1541–1548.

25. Rosati A, Tomassini A, Pollo B, Ambrosi C, Schwarz A, Padovani A, et al. Epilepsy in cerebral glioma: timing of appearance and histological correlations. J. Neurooncol. 2009 July;93:395–400.

26. Phan K, Ng W, Lu VM, McDonald KL, Fairhall J, Reddy R, et al. Association between IDH1 and IDH2 mutations and preoperative seizures in patients with low-grade versus high-grade glioma: a systematic review and meta-analysis. World Neurosurg. 2018 March;111:e539–e545.

27. Chen DY, Chen CC, Crawford JR, Wang SG. Tumor-related epilepsy: epidemiology, pathogenesis and management. J. Neurooncol. 2018 August;139:13–21.
28. Chaichana KL, Parker SL, Olivi A, Quinones-Hinojosa A. Long-term seizure outcomes in adult patients undergoing primary resection of malignant brain astrocytomas: clinical article. J. Neurosurg. 2009 August;111:282–292.
29. Chang EF, Potts MB, Keles GE, Lamborn KR, Chang SM, Barbaro NM, et al. Seizure characteristics and control following resection in 332 patients with low-grade gliomas. J. Neurosurg. 2008 February;108:227–235.
30. Villanueva V, Saiz-Diaz R, Toledo M, Piera A, Mauri JA, Rodriguez-Uranga JJ, et al. NEOPLASM study: real-life use of lacosamide in patients with brain tumor-related epilepsy. Epilepsy Behav. 2016 December;65:25–32.
31. Aronica E, Ciusani E, Coppola A, Costa C, Russo E, Salmaggi A, et al. Epilepsy and brain tumors: two sides of the same coin. J. Neurol. Sci. 2023 March 15;446:120584.
32. Lee PY, Wei YT, Chao KC, Chu CN, Chung WH, Wang TH. Anti-epileptic drug use during adjuvant chemo-radiotherapy is associated with poorer survival in patients with glioblastoma: a nationwide population-based cohort study. J. Cancer Res. Ther. 2024 April 1;20:555–562.
33. Rimmer B, Balla M, Dutton L, Williams S, Araujo-Soares V, Gallagher P, et al. Barriers and facilitators to self-management in people living with a lower-grade glioma. J. Cancer Surviv. 2024 March 21. doi: 10.1007/s11764-024-01572-9 (online ahead of print)
34. Rimmer B, Bolnykh I, Dutton L, Lewis J, Burns R, Gallagher P, et al. Health-related quality of life in adults with low-grade gliomas: a systematic review. Qual. Life Res. 2023 March;32:625–651.
35. Danfors T, Ribom D, Berntsson SG, Smits A. Epileptic seizures and survival in early disease of grade 2 gliomas. Eur. J. Neurol. 2009 July;16:823–831.

Psychosocial Consequences of Acquired Epilepsy

8

8.1 QUALITY OF LIFE

Being a complication to another brain disease, acquired epilepsy often arises in an already challenging medical situation. The patient may be in rehabilitation after the first brain disease and epilepsy complicates an already difficult situation. Plans made for a path back to work and daily living may suffer. Naturally, epilepsy also has an impact even in the absence of perceptible sequelae after the brain disorder. Qualitative research suggests that epilepsy arising midlife may lead to psychosocial challenges that are distinct from epilepsy arising in early adulthood or later with regards to altered life plans, including career, family life, and so forth.[1] There may be a need to revise rehabilitation goals. In this instance it is not uncommon for coping strategies to fail, at least initially. If the epilepsy provider is ready for these reactions, they can sometimes be made easier to deal with. Reassurance that acquired epilepsy is common and that it can be treated successfully is often helpful.

That epilepsy can reduce quality of life after various brain disorders has been demonstrated numerous times; for instance after stroke,[2] traumatic brain injury,[3] brain infections,[4,5] and brain tumors.[6] There is little research on the impact of epilepsy and/or seizures specifically on quality of life in dementia and autoimmune encephalitis but little reason to assume major differences from the other etiologies, and expert opinion or guidelines highlight the importance of epilepsy management in these conditions.[7,8]

Importantly, absence of seizure freedom is in itself associated with poor health-related quality of life. This underlines the importance of pursuing seizure freedom in patients with previous brain disease just as ambitiously as in other epilepsy, while monitoring for side effects and revising therapy as necessary. In refractory cases, epilepsy specialist consultation is almost always advisable.

DOI: 10.1201/9781003501404-8

8.2 COGNITION AND SLEEP

Brain disorders and epilepsy both increases the risk of cognitive impairment, as described in the previous chapters. In all acquired epilepsies, be it after stroke, trauma, tumors, infection, or inflammation, there is a high likelihood of cognitive symptoms like fatigue or other neuropsychological deficits. The difficulties may not be obvious to the patient or even to their families, so neuropsychological testing may be beneficial. Such formal tests of memory, attention, and endurance can help map out cognitive difficulties and guide support.

The cognitive deficits may have psychosocial consequences. Working capacity or ability to participate in family activity can be reduced. Occupational therapist assessment or equivalent can be of value, and sometimes using the results of neuropsychological tests to suggest strategies at home or at work can reduce the impact of the cognitive difficulties. There are digital and non-digital tools for memory assistance, scheduling, and the like.

In many health systems, rehabilitation after a brain insult like stroke, infection, and trauma is an intense inpatient period followed by outpatient visits, ending with discharge. The extent of rehabilitation varies with the availability of rehabilitation services or insurance status of the patient. If rehabilitation is limited or absent, cognitive sequelae may be overlooked. Epilepsy may be the one remaining condition giving the patient regular health care contacts outside of primary care, and in follow-up of epilepsy after brain disorders it is often helpful to be on the lookout for cognitive deficits. Typical examples include persons with traumatic brain injury or treated encephalitis, where cognitive problems can become evident only after return to normal daily activities.

Sleep is epilepsy after brain disorders is an area in need of more research. Poor sleep can be a consequence of several brain lesions and is often also reported in patients without demonstrated brain lesion—like autoimmune encephalitis.[7] Poor sleep decreases quality of life and is also associated with an increased risk of seizures in several forms of epilepsy, but this effect is probably smaller in focal epilepsies than in generalized forms.[9] Whether improved quality of sleep in epilepsy after brain lesions can have an impact on seizure control is an area for future research.

8.3 IMPACT ON REHABILITATION

The impact of epilepsy on rehabilitation after brain diseases is attracting increasing interest. There are methodological problems with disentangling the epilepsy from severity of the initial insult, since more severe stroke, trauma, infection, and so on are risk factors for epilepsy. Nonetheless, it seems intuitive that better seizure control and fewer side effects of medications would be favorable for rehabilitation, and indeed that is what the literature seems to indicate. One review summarized the field as follows: "Overall, a majority of studies suggest that LS and recurrent seizures hamper long-term neurologic outcome after stroke, but several methodologic limitations

TABLE 8.1   Studies on the Association of Poststroke Seizures/Epilepsy with Poor Functional Outcome after Stroke

ISCHEMIC STROKE AND MIXED	N	N EPILEPSY	UNIVARIATE	MULTIVARIATE
Jung et al. 2012[10]	805	18	no association	no association
Bentes et al. 2017[11]	151	23	worse outcome	worse outcome
Creutzfeldt et al. 2014[12]	55	25	worse outcome	
Paolucci et al. 1997[13]	306	46		no association
Arntz et al. 2013[14]	537	54	worse outcome	worse outcome
ICH				
Rossi et al. 2013[15]	325	31	worse outcome	
Biffi et al. 2017[16]	872	79	worse outcome	no association

prevent any definite conclusion on this important issue."[17] Apart from the severity of the stroke itself, there may be other confounders. For instance, the authors of a study that found worse outcome in patients with ICH and epilepsy in univariate analysis (HR 1.8), but not when correcting for imaging characteristics, noted that the association may be partly confounded by small vessel disease.[16]

Epilepsy after stroke and trauma has been the most extensively studied with regards to functional outcome. In a multivariate analysis, poststroke epilepsy was independently associated with poor outcome after rehabilitation after cerebral infarction in more than 500 young stroke patients, as assessed by mRS.[14] Of note, there are also negative studies, finding that poststroke epilepsy did not negatively impact rehabilitation (Table 8.1).[15, 33] In ICH and post-traumatic epilepsy, some neurosurgical units administer primary ASM prophylaxis in patients that have not had seizures, thereby allowing study of the impact on ASM on rehabilitation. The results are not clear, but at least older ASMs like phenytoin could have a negative impact on rehabilitation.[18] It is not certain that this extends to levetiracetam, but theoretically all ASMs can have tiredness and cognitive side effects that are probably not beneficial for rehabilitation. Just as important as avoidance of side effects is of course the treatment of seizures.

8.4 DRIVING

Loss of driving privileges is one of the more severe effects of epilepsy from a psychosocial perspective and can in many countries contribute to both stigma and isolation of persons with epilepsy. There are often legal requirements of reporting to the driving authorities that put strains on the patient–doctor relation, depending on whether it is the responsibility of patients or doctors to report the presence of epilepsy to the authorities. In the European Union, the general rule is that a first seizure needs to be followed by six months seizure freedom before driving a car/motorcycle. In cases of epilepsy a seizure means that driving of a car/motorcycle is not allowed until 12 months have passed without a new seizure. For heavy vehicles, taxi, or equivalent, the times required are much longer. In the US, regulations and observation time vary between states.

The seizure-free observation times are meant to bring the annual seizure relapse risk below 20%. It is important to recognize that a first seizure after a brain insult in many cases indicates a higher risk of recurrence than after an unprovoked seizure in the absence of a previous brain disorder. A longer period of abstinence is probably required. In some instances, like after stroke or severe trauma, epilepsy can sometimes be diagnosed already after a first seizure.

Although driving issues can complicate the patient–physician relationship, it is vital to adhere to local reporting laws and remember to counsel the patient regarding driving. Accidents can be severe, and insurance may not always be valid if driving has occurred against medical advice. In patients with other brain disorders it is also important not to forget other aspects of fitness to drive than the time since the last seizure. Cognitive problems or visual field defects are the two most commonly encountered barriers to return to driving encountered in patients with previous brain disorders.

CASE 8.1 Return to Driving

A 65-year-old female sustains a traumatic brain injury with contusions in the right parietal and temporal lobes, suffers an acute symptomatic seizure while in the hospital, and is started on levetiracetam, which is withdrawn after three months. Three weeks later she suffers two focal to bilateral tonic-clonic seizures, is diagnosed with post-traumatic epilepsy, and is restarted on ASM therapy. She remains seizure free for one year and at a follow-up visit expresses excitement on soon being able to drive again once she has been seizure free for one year. Review of the records indicates substantial cognitive problems during the rehabilitation after the traumatic brain injury, and review of the radiology puts the contusions at least in the area of the optic radiation on the right.

Comment: This vignette illustrates that seizure freedoms may not be the only aspect to consider when evaluating fitness to drive. In this case, it may be suitable with cognitive testing and formal visual field examination.

8.5 SEIZURE-RELATED RISKS

In addition to driving, seizures can be dangerous if they arise in the wrong situation (Table 8.2). Most quality systems for epilepsy care indicate that caregivers should advise patients on seizure-related risks. Typical situations to mention are heights, swimming, and dangerous machinery. Falls are one of the most commonly sustained seizure-related injuries, and swimming can be very dangerous if one is unconscious. Importantly, supervision of a person with epilepsy needs to be constant and individual; drownings at school outings

TABLE 8.2   Important Seizure-Related Risks That Need to Be Discussed

Driving
Heights
Swimming/activities near water
Dangerous machinery/activities
SUDEP

have occurred with several teachers watching a group of children—it is very easy to miss one person disappearing. It is also important not to underestimate the weight of a person with a seizure; ideally, the supervised person should not be swimming in greater depths than would allow a rescuer to stand with the feet on the bottom should a seizure happen. Giving correct advice can be a balancing act, and it is important to avoid overprotection and increasing stigma. All risk assessment needs to be individualized—patients need to consider what their seizures entail and what the consequences would be in different circumstances. A Swedish population-based study found the risks of accidents, including falls and drowning, to be increased in persons with epilepsy.[19] The risk was most elevated in the first years after the diagnosis, underlining the need to give advice on seizure-related risks early on.

8.5.1 SUDEP

Sudden unexpected death in epilepsy is a difficult area to counsel patients and family about and is often overlooked. International guidelines try to change the situation and stipulate that health services are to inform persons with epilepsy about the risk of SUDEP.[20] Application of this advice varies across countries and cultures, but in general, it is helpful to inform about but emphasize the low risk for most patients. Without information from health services, patients may well end up trusting and being worried by information online. The risk of SUDEP is about 1/1000 patient years.[21] The risk is closely tied to the frequency of tonic-clonic seizures, which illustrates the importance of adherence to ASM prescriptions. In fact, ASM treatment may help also when it does not completely prevent seizures: an interesting meta-analysis showed that the SUDEP frequency was lower in patients with active substance compared to placebo in randomized controlled trials of focal epilepsy.[22] Of particular interest in the field of epilepsy in other brain disorders is that structural epilepsy etiology was identified in one study as a SUDEP risk factor.[23]

8.6 WORKING LIFE

Epilepsy can have an impact on work. There may be formal restrictions on driving, and employers may feel concern for health and safety. The patient may need support from a work counselor. The loss of ability to work is often perceived as one of the major impacts of having epilepsy.

8.6.1 Employment

Epilepsy is somewhat more common in persons of low socioeconomic standing,[24,25] which is probably because low level of education and low income are statistically associated with other risk factors of epilepsy—like poor cardiovascular health and higher risk of traumatic brain injury. That low socioeconomic position is correlated with increased prevalence of disease is not unique for epilepsy; the same association is seen, for instance, in cancer and cardiovascular disease. Importantly, some studies from the US as well as Denmark and Sweden, which are welfare states, indicate that the personal economic consequences of developing epilepsy, like low income and unemployment, can be greater for persons of low socioeconomic standing.[24–29] The reason for the phenomenon is unknown, but heightened awareness can be needed if a person who already is in a precarious position on the labor market develops epilepsy. Additional counselling may be helpful with regards to employment.

8.6.2 Seizure Frequency and Work

One of the important risk factors for problems at work caused by epilepsy seems to be a high seizure frequency. Stigmatization, seizure-related loss of working hours, and negative stress spirals are some probable explanations. Patients with more seizures are less likely to be able to work and report more problems at work than patients who are seizure free.[27–29] ASM polytherapy may be an important contributor.

Importantly, there is no one-size-fits-all assessment of fitness to work—some persons with intractable epilepsy can work full time. In time, medically refractory epilepsy tends to lead to part-time work or retreat from the labor market. Conversely, seizure freedom does not automatically mean that a person with epilepsy does not have difficulties in his or her working life; side effects of ASMs, fear of seizures, cognitive problems from the epilepsy or the previous brain disorder causing epilepsy, or psychiatric comorbidities are important reasons. Patients undergoing epilepsy surgery clearly illustrate the difficulty in relating seizure frequency to working capacity. Some patients are not able to return to work despite achieving a very successful surgery outcome, often because of cognitive problems or other ASM side effects.[32]

8.6.3 Nature of Difficulties at Work

Problems at work can be both physical and psychosocial (Table 8.3). Frequently encountered problems include feelings of exclusion, restrictions on activities, stress because of time lost due to seizures, stress because of reduced working capacity caused by ASM, side effects, and stigma.[28,29] Medical advice can be needed on sick leave, rehabilitation, and adaptation of work environment from a health and safety perspective. The activity limitation imposed by seizures must be assessed on an individual basis, but risk situations are typically heights, water, and dangerous machinery. For office work, special attention needs to be directed towards the level of stress. Stress is sometimes a seizure

TABLE 8.3   Problems in the Working Life Reported by Persons with Epilepsy in Qualitative Studies

Stigma
Driving license requirements
Loss of working time because of seizures
Worse performance because of seizures or side effects
Having to avoid certain tasks for fear of seizures
Ashamed after seizures at work

precipitant, but more importantly reduced working capacity due to fear of seizures, ASM side effects, or the psychological impact of being diagnosed with epilepsy can lead to burnout. A gradual return to work is often advisable.

Whether a patient should disclose epilepsy at work is sometimes brought up in contact with epilepsy services. The answer is difficult, and the advisable action probably varies between patients, countries, and cultures. Some European studies indicate that persons with epilepsy wish to disclose their condition—so that co-workers can assist in case of a seizure and to avoid the feeling of withholding an important aspect of their life. These qualitative findings also indicate that there can be a sense of "hiding" epilepsy if it is not being disclosed.[30] This is countered by the fear of stigmatization and not being treated the same as before. There is no clear advice from a medical point of view, other than that the patient should obviously follow legal requirements related to certain jobs to report changes in health status, and that management often needs to be informed to be able to create a safe work environment.

8.7 FAMILY LIFE

Acquired epilepsy can disrupt family life. Just like in all epilepsy, psychosocial problems like divorce and financial difficulties are more common after diagnosis. Families are often supportive and go to great lengths to facilitate return to normal life, but patients may nonetheless report feeling guilty over having yet another health condition. Counselling can often help.

8.8 PSYCHIATRIC COMORBIDITIES

In addition to cognitive sequelae and seizures, patients with epilepsy with or without another brain disorder may have psychiatric comorbidities; most commonly depression and anxiety. Recognition and treatment of such disorders, whether reactive or not, may significantly help. There are epidemiological associations between epilepsy and depression, as well as epilepsy and very severe psychiatric symptoms such as suicidality. Importantly, the relationships seems bidirectional—suicidality is a risk factor for epilepsy and vice versa.[31] Pathophysiological explanations are currently not entirely clear, but the association could for instance indicate that mechanisms inducing depression also underlie epileptogenesis. However, most ASMs have a black box warning for suicidality, which needs to be monitored for when starting an ASM.

What health care provider actually manages depression or anxiety depends on the local care structure, but from an epilepsy point of view the important message is that epilepsy should not prevent adequate treatment of psychiatric comorbidities. Fear of interactions between antidepressants and ASMs or that antidepressants can cause or aggravate seizures may be obstacles in providing good psychiatric care. Many such fears are based on misconceptions.[31] Concerns about worsening epilepsy with psychiatric medications or vice versa can generally be resolved through consultations between involved specialties.

8.9 CARE PATHWAYS

Although epilepsy is a common complication of brain diseases, care systems sometimes fail to adequately identify and treat patients. Poststroke epilepsy is the most researched area in this regard. Even in countries like Sweden, with free health care and a relatively equal income distribution, patients with poststroke epilepsy often receive suboptimal epilepsy care, presumably because they are not cared for by doctors trained in epilepsy. The most common scenario is that a patient has a first seizure and is put on levetiracetam or another ASM in the emergency room. Soon, follow-up is shifted to primary care or other non-epilepsy providers, where occasional seizures may be perceived not as treatment failure prompting a dose increase or other therapy revision but as a normal state of affairs. Conversely, side effects of ASMs may be misinterpreted as sequelae of the original brain disease.

The aforementioned suboptimal care pathways probably underlie the common perception that acquired epilepsy is easy to treat when longitudinal studies in fact suggest that it is not very different from other epilepsies. That a patient is never seen again after being started on an ASM may not mean that he or she is doing well. Judging from the present literature, a substantial proportion of patients with brain disease will develop medically refractory epilepsy. For optimal epilepsy care, patients with acquired epilepsy need to be seen by epilepsy services and treated in the same manner as all other patients: titration of a carefully selected ASM until seizure freedom or intolerable side effects with therapy revision in case of treatment failure.

REFERENCES

1. Kilinc S, van Wersch A, Campbell C, Guy A. The experience of living with adult-onset epilepsy. Epilepsy Behav. 2017 August;73: 189–196.
2. Winter Y, Daneshkhah N, Galland N, Kotulla I, Kruger A, Groppa S. Health-related quality of life in patients with poststroke epilepsy. Epilepsy Behav. 2018 March;80: 303–306.

3. Gugger JJ, Kennedy E, Panahi S, Tate DF, Roghani A, Van Cott AC, et al. Multimodal quality of life assessment in post-9/11 veterans with epilepsy: impact of drug resistance, traumatic brain injury, and comorbidity. Neurology. 2022 April 26;98:e1761–e1770.

4. de Almeida SM, Gurjao SA. Quality of life assessment in patients with neurocysticercosis. J. Community Health. 2011 August;36: 624–630.

5. Zapata WR, Yang SY, Bustos JA, Gonzales I, Saavedra H, Guzman C, et al. Quality of life in patients with symptomatic epilepsy due to neurocysticercosis. Epilepsy Behav. 2022 June;131:108668.

6. Rimmer B, Bolnykh I, Dutton L, Lewis J, Burns R, Gallagher P, et al. Health-related quality of life in adults with low-grade gliomas: a systematic review. Qual. Life Res. 2023 March;32: 625–651.

7. Turcano P, Day GS. Life after autoantibody-mediated encephalitis: optimizing follow-up and management in recovering patients. Curr. Opin. Neurol. 2022 June 1;35: 415–422.

8. Frederiksen KS, Cooper C, Frisoni GB, Frolich L, Georges J, Kramberger MG, et al. A European Academy of Neurology guideline on medical management issues in dementia. Eur. J. Neurol. 2020 October;27: 1805–1820.

9. Grigg-Damberger MM, Ralls F. Sleep disorders in adults with epilepsy: past, present, and future directions. Curr. Opin. Pulm. Med. 2014 November;20: 542–549.

10. Jung S, Schindler K, Findling O, Mono ML, Fischer U, Gralla J, et al. Adverse effect of early epileptic seizures in patients receiving endovascular therapy for acute stroke. Stroke J. Cereb. Circ. 2012 June;43: 1584–1590.

11. Bentes C, Peralta AR, Martins H, Casimiro C, Morgado C, Franco AC, et al. Seizures, electroencephalographic abnormalities, and outcome of ischemic stroke patients. Epilepsia Open. 2017 December;2: 441–452.

12. Creutzfeldt CJ, Tirschwell DL, Kim LJ, Schubert GB, Longstreth WT Jr, Becker KJ. Seizures after decompressive hemicraniectomy for ischaemic stroke. J. Neurol. Neurosurg. Psychiatry. 2014 July;85: 721–725.

13. Paolucci S, Silvestri G, Lubich S, Pratesi L, Traballesi M, Gigli GL. Poststroke late seizures and their role in rehabilitation of inpatients. Epilepsia. 1997 March;38: 266–270.

14. Arntz RM, Maaijwee NA, Rutten-Jacobs LC, Schoonderwaldt HC, Dorresteijn LD, van Dijk EJ, et al. Epilepsy after TIA or stroke in young patients impairs long-term functional outcome: the FUTURE study. Neurology. 2013 November 26;81: 1907–1913.

15. Rossi C, De Herdt V, Dequatre-Ponchelle N, Henon H, Leys D, Cordonnier C. Incidence and predictors of late seizures in intracerebral hemorrhages. Stroke J. Cereb. Circ. 2013 June;44: 1723–1725.

16. Biffi A, Rattani A, Anderson CD, Ayres AM, Gurol EM, Greenberg SM, et al. Delayed seizures after intracerebral haemorrhage. Brain J. Neurol. 2016 October;139: 2694–2705.

17. Ryvlin P, Montavont A, Nighoghossian N. Optimizing therapy of seizures in stroke patients. Neurology. 2006 December 26;67:S3–S9.

18. Koch S, Sung G. AEDs after ICH: preventing the prophylaxis. Neurology. 2017 January 3;88: 15–16.

19. Mahler B, Carlsson S, Andersson T, Tomson T. Risk for injuries and accidents in epilepsy: a prospective population-based cohort study. Neurology. 2018 February 27;90:e779–e789.

20. Harden C, Tomson T, Gloss D, Buchhalter J, Cross JH, Donner E, et al. Practice guideline summary: sudden unexpected death in epilepsy incidence rates and risk factors: report of the Guideline Development, Dissemination, and Implementation Subcommittee of the American Academy of Neurology and the American Epilepsy Society. Neurology. 2017 April 25;88: 1674–1680.

21. Sveinsson O, Andersson T, Mattsson P, Carlsson S, Tomson T. Clinical risk factors in SUDEP: a nationwide population-based case-control study. Neurology. 2020 January 28;94:e419–e429.

22. Ryvlin P, Cucherat M, Rheims S. Risk of sudden unexpected death in epilepsy in patients given adjunctive antiepileptic treatment for refractory seizures: a meta-analysis of placebo-controlled randomised trials. Lancet Neurol. 2011 November;10: 961–968.

23. Sveinsson O, Andersson T, Carlsson S, Tomson T. Type, etiology, and duration of epilepsy as risk factors for SUDEP: further analyses of a population-based case-control study. Neurology. 2023 November 27;101:e2257–e2265.

24. Andersson K, Ozanne A, Tranberg AE, Chaplin JE, Bolin K, Malmgren K, et al. Socioeconomic outcome and access to care in adults with epilepsy in Sweden: a nationwide cohort study. Seizure. 2019 December 3;74: 71–76.

25. Steer S, Pickrell WO, Kerr MP, Thomas RH. Epilepsy prevalence and socioeconomic deprivation in England. Epilepsia. 2014 October;55: 1634–1641.

26. Jennum P, Sabers A, Christensen J, Ibsen R, Kjellberg J. Welfare consequences for people with epilepsy and their partners: a matched nationwide study in Denmark. Seizure. 2017 July;49: 17–24.

27. Lindsten H, Stenlund H, Edlund C, Forsgren L. Socioeconomic prognosis after a newly diagnosed unprovoked epileptic seizure in adults: a population-based case-control study. Epilepsia. 2002 October;43: 1239–1250.

28. Chaplin JE, Wester A, Tomson T. Factors associated with the employment problems of people with established epilepsy. Seizure. 1998 August;7: 299–303.

29. Chung K, Liu Y, Ivey SL, Huang D, Chung C, Guo W, et al. Quality of life in epilepsy (QOLIE): insights about epilepsy and support groups from people with epilepsy (San Francisco Bay Area, USA). Epilepsy Behav. 2012 June;24: 256–263.

30. Elliott N, Pembroke S, Quirke M, Pender N, Higgins A. Disclosure strategies in adults with epilepsy when telling, "I have epilepsy": the How2tell study. Epilepsia. 2019 October;60: 2048–2059.

31. Kanner AM, Shankar R, Margraf NG, Schmitz B, Ben-Menachem E, Sander JW. Mood disorders in adults with epilepsy: a review of unrecognized facts and common misconceptions. Ann. Gen. Psychiatry. 2024 March 4;23:11.

32. Edelvik A, Flink R, Malmgren K. Prospective and longitudinal long-term employment outcomes after resective epilepsy surgery. Neurology. 2015 October 27;85:1482–1490.

33. De Herdt V, Dumont F, Henon H, Derambure P, Vonck K, Leys D, et al. Early seizures in intracerebral hemorrhage: incidence, associated factors, and outcome. Neurology. 2011 November 15;77: 1794–1800.

Index

Note: Page numbers in *italics* indicate a figure and page numbers in **bold** indicate a table on the corresponding page.